3/6/06
I recently ae
lecture by the
even one "ah ho
you improve your u...
that will be terrific.
Let me know your thoughts!
Love from Judy

THE BEST LITTLE HEALTH BOOK EVER

THE SIMPLE WHYS AND HOWS OF FEELING YOUR BEST EVERY DAY

BY

SUSANNE MORRONE, B.S., CNC

CARTOON ILLUSTRATIONS BY JEFF DOKKEN

Llumina Press

ISBN: 1-932560-83-1
Printed in the United States of America by Llumina Press

This book is not a medical book to diagnose, treat, cure or manage disease. It shares with you the beautiful truth that the gift of good health is within our grasp. When we choose to practice tried and true principles of healthy living, the healing power within is strengthened.

Talk Health. The dreary, never changing tale of mortal maladies is worn and stale.

You cannot charm, or interest, or please by harping on that minor chord, disease.

Say you are well, or all is well with you, And God shall hear your words and make them true.

("Optimism" by Ella Wheeler Wilcox)

DEDICATED TO

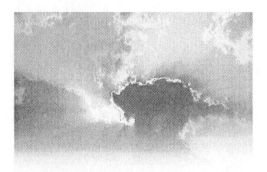

The Master Architect of the awesome universe,
Our Heavenly Father, who designed us with an
innate ability to heal. To Him goes all the praise.

Table of Contents

PART THREE: Feeding the Soul

INTRODUCTION

Growing up in the 20th century, the majority of us were schooled to think health in all its possible aspects was synonymous with "doctor." Not feeling well meant an automatic trek to the all seeing, all knowing person in the white lab coat who would hopefully identify the problem and hand us the cure. This auto pilot response somehow made the doctor solely responsible for the state of our health.. Although this often is a frustrating and worry-ridden exercise, we realize we may have too little knowledge to correct the situation ourselves.

Each day we're bombarded with an avalanche of fragmented health information. The evening news entices us with announcements to watch and learn what are the best foods to eat, the ultimate diets, the hottest supplements and new medical developments which will cure disease and revolutionize health care as we know it. Infomercials would have us believe that absolute health is to be found in one magic pill, potion, lotion, contraption or miracle procedure. Without a definitive road map, we struggle on in confusion to try to get to our destination and may never reach it.

When the desire to see what we can do ourselves emerges, we turn to the untold volumes of books written on virtually every aspect of health. Combing library shelves and bookstores, we find many technical and challenging reads. Natural health books promote taking better care of ourselves. They offer general or specific guidelines on what foods, supplements and modalities improve a particular health challenge. Many well-researched authors present the benefits of a single nutrient or method, and the reader often interprets this singular item to be the panacea for all his/her ills. This is not a far-fetched assumption. Health professionals themselves who've gravitated to one therapy or product can become narrow in scope and purport their remedy as the definitive answer. For the person becoming weary in the quest for appropriate answers and desirable results, these accolades may resound as just one more empty promise to better health.

For almost twenty years, I've spoken to countless school age students up through senior citizens who ask for a book to explain why and how natural health works and possibly how to get started. My search to find one straightforward, easy to understand book that illuminates the whole picture did not bring results. Seeing the considerable interest from people of all ages who want clarity spurred me on to write "The Best Little Health Book Ever." It offers the simple whys and hows of feeling your best every day. It will appeal to your common sense and instill an increased awareness of the necessity of a complete, balanced approach. The way to attain your health goals will no longer be elusive. You're not going to read a new concept, something I developed because I'm a genius nor one brought about by high-tech scientific innovation. Actually, wise King Solomon, King of ancient Israel, brought to our attention in Ecclesiastes that "What has been will be again, what has been done will be done again; there is nothing new under the sun. Is there anything of which one can say, 'Look, there is something new!' It was here already, long ago; it was here before our time." Each new generation rearranges things, combine things not combined in exactly the same manner as before, but always starts with what's already here. There may be cloning, stem cell regeneration and foreskin grafts, but let me know when someone takes an empty test tube and creates life. Then, I'll be impressed. Thomas Edison, known for his outspoken wisdom, said: "Until man duplicates a blade of grass, nature can laugh at his so-called scientific knowledge... It's obvious that we don't know one millionth of one percent about anything."

Many in the medical community driven by ego and prejudices, still discredit herbs and food supplements as ineffective at best, even possibly "dangerous." "They can cause catastrophic consequences!.," I was recently told by one staunch medical man. The typical comment you'll hear is that "Natural supplement products have no double-blind studies to back them up", or "They do not have the rubber stamp of scientific soundness." (Although this may have been true years ago, we see an explosion of scientific research heralding the nutrients in foods and benefits of supplements.) Discrediting comments instill fear and skepticism in the uninformed. Are we motivated enough to get the full story, or figure these things are unproven and unsafe? We can decide to pass on vitamins, herbs and other supplements, opt for nothing to change and the same old results.

Two incidents stand out in my mind. Each different, yet both spawned from fear. Several years ago, a new client of mine frantically called me. After calming her down, I asked why she was so fearful. Someone she just met heard it through the grapevine that a person died from drinking carrot juice. This was told to her just minutes after she had enjoyed a freshly-juiced carrot, apple, ginger combination at a Wild Oats Market. Suddenly, carrots were on par in her mind with hemlock and toadstools. I know truth is stranger than fiction, and anything is possible in the most unusual of circumstances. The gentle carrot could be intentionally or unintentionally poisoned by man's toxic chemicals. I told her if she ran out in front of a fast-moving truck carrying a cargo of carrots it probably would. We both laughed, talked about what each of us wanted to accomplish that day.

On another occasion, I was asked to take a call from a woman who had just finished her last chemotherapy treatment and was told nothing more could be done for her. The cancer was out of control. With extreme trepidation, she asked, "Do you think it would hurt me to take some B vitamins?" It is sad to think we willingly undergo conventional treatments without questioning consequences far worse perhaps than any disease would do in terms of cellular damage, degraded immune function and imbalanced body systems. Yet, we fear what a vitamin may do to our precious life. My heart went out to her.

Empirical evidence is there for millenniums on the effectiveness of herbal medicine in promoting healthy living. Scientific knowledge of herbs has been accumulating rapidly for the past 100 years. People who took herbs as medicine and ate the bounty from their gardens may not have known about proanthocyanidins molecules, sulforaphane, ellagic acid, tocotrineols, zeaxanthin or indole 3-carbinols, but they did enjoy longer, healthier lives. For us to obtain good health, we must use an approach that is firmly founded on the understanding of the healing power of the living body. It is the science and art of giving the body what it needs naturally-- proper food, rest, sleep, fresh air, sunlight, pure water, exercise, relaxation, cleanliness, work, play, positive mental processes, and food for the soul or spirit. Exercise by itself brings some benefit just as a good diet will. But piecemeal input will not be sufficient to build good health. It takes a superb comprehensive approach of balanced, wholesome living. This is not a system of medicine nor of healing arts. It does not cure; it enables the power within to cure. It supports and respects how this is accomplished.

We pay too high a price to be ignorant to the true causes of disease, health and healing. The physical body, mind, emotions and spirit are all intertwined. When something is awry, it affects the whole. How can it possibly be advantageous to isolate individual body parts or symptoms? When we do so we usually settle for disappointing, often temporary results. Without understanding, we insist our symptoms and complaints be addressed quickly with symptomatic treatment-- an antihistamine to dry up a runny nose, a steroid cream to stop the itchy rash, an antacid to cool the burning stomach, an analgesic to bring down a fever.... and so it goes. Is this not "disease management" instead of true prevention? We're never just a stomach ache or sore throat. For these problems to surface, they must have a cause. We are not low or deficient in the drug we take for the symptom. If we fail to question, we can keep playing the same old tune on a worn out fiddle.

Longed-for, lasting results come from addressing the cause. Until we recognize this, we'll keep putting our bodies through much unnecessary suffering, actually postponing health problems. These problems may rear their ugly heads later with more severity. Thomas Edison caught the vision of this when he made one of his most famous quotes on health: "The doctor of the future will give no medicine but will interest his patients in the care of the human frame, in diet and in the cause and prevention of disease. The physician of tomorrow will be the nutritionist of today." Yes, its nice to know that scientific research is beginning to catch up with empirical evidence. In the meantime, amidst all of this discovery, we should cultivate a desire to take more responsibility for our health, learn what truly builds it, make a commitment to get well, and apply the principles of healthy living on a day to day basis.

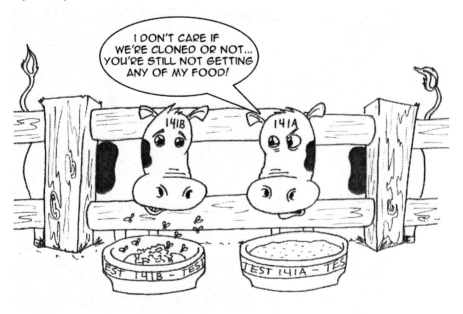

PART ONE:
WHAT'S WRONG WITH US ANYWAY?

CHAPTER ONE

LEARN FROM THE PAST AND GROW

> Dwell not on the past.
> Use it to illustrate a point,
> then leave it behind.
> Nothing really matters
> except what you do now
> in this instant of time.
> From this moment onward
> you can be an entirely
> different person,
> filled with love and understanding
> ready with an outstretched hand,
> uplifted and positive
> in every thought and deed.

From "God Spoke to Me" by Eileen Caddy

It's a 21st Century Day...

6:20 a.m. That blaring alarm shocks us out of deep sleep. Walk sluggishly to the kitchen, brew some caffeine or decaf. Light up a cigarette; haven't been able to quit.

6:30 a.m. Into the bathroom for a chlorinated, perhaps heavy-metal laden shower. Shampoo and scrub with an assortment of chemicals, rub aluminum deodorant under the arms, use a vast assortment of chemicalized creams, lotions and sprays. Apply cosmetics containing toxic chemicals on the skin. Blow dry hair and get dressed.

7:15 a.m. Pop a sugary toaster strudel in the micro and decide between a quick coffee or cold cola for the ride. Gulp down the strudel on the way to the car. Got to pick up donuts for the office and stop for gas.

7:20 a.m. Pull into the gas station. Wait impatiently in line to pay. Look at wrist watch to check the time. Pump the gas-- Ughhh!!, the aroma of gasoline. Wipe the gas and oily black film off your hands. Check the time again. Pull out into heavy traffic and begin the stress-filled drive to work.

7:50 a.m. The driver to your left speeds up, uses no signal, cuts across your lane and the next, to turn right at the intersection. "Where did you learn how to drive? #@!!*+??%#!!!." Heave a sigh and turn on the radio to catch the news. Shut it off, just more stress.

8:00 a.m. Made it to the parking lot, just in time. Power walk to the entrance. Grab a coffee and donut. Go to work station. Experience a variety of toxins depending upon type of work-- perhaps just high noise intrusion, emf's (low-level electromagnetic frequencies) from the computer monitor.

10:15 a.m. Take a cigarette break and visit the vending machine. Gulp down a can of soda with 12 tsp. of sugar or a "diet" brand with artificial sweeteners, dyes and miscellaneous other chemicals. Those peanut butter crackers look good, too.

12:00 noon. Rush out the door to a fast food restaurant drive-through. Light up a cigarette since the line is so long. Check the time. Take the hydrogenated fat burger, fries and soft drink back to work. Gulp it hurriedly, have to meet deadline.

2:30 p.m. Yawning, sleepiness and fatigue set in. Take another vending machine break for a jolt of energy. See if any donuts left.

3:00 p.m. Take a pill for a headache and perhaps an antacid. This work load has to lighten up!

6:00 p.m. Leave work and stop at the dry cleaners. Put the clothes in the back seat to outgas vapors of toluene, benzene, formaldehyde and other chemicals. Wait in heavy traffic, anxiously, while muttering under your breath. Weave in and out of traffic to avoid the slow drivers.

7:00 p.m. Hang the dry-cleaned clothes in the closet. Pop a "mean cuisine" in the micro. Have another cigarette. Notice some ants crawling on the counter. Spray them with insecticide. Pet and feed the cat, no time to wash hands and gulp down dinner in front of TV (Phone interrupts-- friends coming by later.)

7:25 p.m. Clean the litter box, take out the trash and run the vacuum cleaner. Might as well get one more use out of the dirty bag. Dust, bacteria and animal dander fills the air. Notice the "funky smell" and plug in the flora air freshener containing chemicals that deaden the nerve endings in your nostrils so the odor is undetectable.

7:40 p.m. Have a cold, refreshing beer. Take a quick shower. Use the same chemicalized body products as in early a.m. Get dressed, put on a pot of coffee, defrost a frozen dessert in the micro.

8:00 p.m. Company arrives. Order a pizza. Drink a cola with pizza. Have some defrosted dessert, ice cream and coffee.

9:30 p.m. Have heartburn, take an antacid.

10:45 p.m. Company leaves. Take an aspirin for that lingering headache. Clean up dishes and take out trash. Get ready for bed. Watch a little more TV.

11:30 p.m. Really tired. Turn off lights and TV. Sink into bed, the pillow feels good.

12:15 a.m. Can't sleep, take a sleeping aid.

3:30 a.m. Wake up and go to the bathroom. Back to bed. Dead tired, fall asleep.

6:30 a.m. Rise and shine. It's another day!

Sound familiar? This is a fairly typical day for many working people. Why are we doing this to ourselves? We fastidiously fuel our cars for optimum performance. We pay little attention to fueling our bodies, then wonder why our tires go flat, our batteries run low, we get cobwebs in our exhaust pipes, we spit, sputter, cough and choke and willingly have major parts replaced. And, these overhauls get quite expensive. Are we not worth far more than the cars we drive? We may own five to ten cars in a lifetime, but we only get one physical human body per lifetime. That's reason enough to take good care of it.

Back to School

Graduation --whether it's ahead of you or merely a sweet memory-- is always a time for serious reflection upon all that you've learned, and all you hope to accomplish in the future. Each graduate overflows with expectations of achieving full potential, while making an indelible mark in the world. It was no different for me, and I was filled with the heady excitement of future promise. As class valedictorian, I was given first choice of the three topics offered for our high school commencement speeches. As soon as I heard "Education Influences the World", I wanted the privilege to develop a speech to look at the earth from a higher, more meaningful, perspective. This for me was a weighty and solemn assignment which I attacked with great enthusiasm. Well-chosen words could remove national boundaries and prejudices that separate people, and mankind might then become one entity continually faced with choices.

What I saw was that first and foremost, man has developed the technology to heroically save many lives, while at the same time, acquiring the ability to destroy countless others in heinous holocausts. We are fortunate to have had many millenniums from which to learn, but unfortunately, it seems we haven't learned much. The question is, when will we relent from the dire consequences of short-sightedness and greed in order to use our lives in caring for this earth and for each other? Individually we all must take a stand. We must search for accurate knowledge rather than be deluded by falsehoods and deceptions which bring devastation.

This graduation event is shared with you since it does have a bearing on the subject of building and maintaining health. Education holds the key to enjoying the precious life we have and the gift of good health. We must cut through all the teachings, philosophies and -isms to find life-giving truth. This search goes hand in hand with assuming personal responsibility for our health which is too precious to relinquish to someone else's decision-making process.

Blessings In Change

On July 29, 1997, I received a most cherished letter from one of my clients in Albuquerque. It means so much to me that his health had greatly improved, and it also brought back important early thoughts I had tucked away and forgotten. I'll just highlight for you one paragraph from this letter:

"As a direct result of the program Susanne instituted for me, I have achieved a level of health previously unknown to me.

I am a lifelong, steroid dependent asthmatic. Via a program of dietary changes and vitamins, minerals and herbs, my asthma has virtually disappeared.

Over the past two years while working with Susanne and my doctor, I have eliminated many prescription medications. To breathe freely and clearly every minute of every day is an amazing gift.".

Sincerely, Stuart G.

Remembering Years Gone By

As I read those lines, it brought back memories of childhood. The earliest, vivid recollection I have is of peering through the rungs of my crib at the jar of petroleum jelly about a foot and a half away. It was nap time, but there undoubtedly was too much for me to see and think about. Pressing my face against the white rung while stretching and straining my left arm, I was able to seize this object for closer inspection. The lid came off fairly easily, and voila! my artistic flair was born. My right index finger took the rainbow of imaginary colors from that large economy-sized jar and made the most interesting swirls, curves and lines on the wallpaper. Admiring my first mural brought a huge smile to my face. This was art appreciation at its finest. Mother, as I recall, became the unimpressed art critic who did not share in my celebration of accomplishment.

What she did share in was tireless, vigilant care for my weak constitution as infancy was riddled with allergies, chest colds and frequent prescriptions for antibiotics. Long, arduous nights were spent with me lying on my stomach across her lap or cradled in her arms on that creaking green vinyl rocker. I would look up at her so thankful for her loving touch with dark purple circles under my "owl" eyes, exhausted from laboring to breathe. I thought of this and also another specific incident which happened at age four. I was resting on my knees and forearms in bed straining for air. This health situation caused me to do a lot of serious thinking and questioning at a very young age. Wanting comfort at that moment, I asked God to please let me get more air, help my Mom (who was steadfast attending to my needs), and enable me someday to help stop the suffering of others with allergies, asthma and other breathing problems. The thought of Him helping me to bring relief to others was comforting. I lay there thinking about all those possibilities in earnest. Maybe someday..... some way.

Hurrying Up to Wait

My parents took me almost weekly to Dr. Limbert's office for allergy shots. The waiting room was always full, and it seemed like hours before my name was announced. I distinctly remember looking around at all the sad and somber faces. A series of scratch tests determined the source of my allergies to be dust, mold, ragweed, chocolate, grapes and cheese. Chocolate was a culprit causing itchy, red wheals on my skin after eating Hershey Bars and 3 Musketeers. So, instead of those, I was now eating penicillin, Teramyacin, and cherry cough syrup.

I also remember the annual "TB drive" in our grade school. It was a brief, brisk walk past Ruth, the school nurse, who knitted her eyebrows each time she pointed emphatically at a student. She singled out the frail, frazzled or skinny child to be grouped together with all the others who got the point. It meant time off from school for a chest x-ray to determine tuberculosis. I was pointed out two years in a row from the lineup, but fortunately tested negative.

Another similar humiliation was those high-tech, expensive nose filters which my well-meaning, concerned parents bought for me to wear. These consisted of a series of stacked filters in a 1/4 inch metal band shaped to fit inside each nostril. In theory they were a good idea to keep out the dust, mold and ragweed spores. However, try to tell any kid to wear those puppies to school. They were very visible in the bathroom mirror when my head was tilted. So, everyone else obviously could see them. Who wants to leave the comfort of home to face ridicule and name-calling: there goes- "Sue, the human vacuum cleaner"- . Not me! The dust, pollen, and molds had to make the trip through my unenhanced nasal passages, and the filters went into a kitchen drawer. There was also a disgustingly bitter, tiny red pill I was ordered to place under my tongue for easier breathing. They didn't work either since they were stuffed under the mattress and behind the headboard as soon as Mom turned to leave the room. So, it was back to the doctor's waiting room for the next round of innovations.

Growing up in Pennsylvania, we saw some pretty cold winters. Excitement filled the air with each big snowfall, because it meant sledding, building snow forts and snowball fights. With all the layers of clothing, we waddled out the front door twice our normal size, like mummies, and hoped we didn't have to visit the bathroom a few minutes later. One particular winter the roads were plowed, and the snow on each side of the car was higher than the car roof. Driving was reminiscent of laboratory rats finding their way through a maze.

My excitement about winter, unfortunately, was mixed with much apprehension about sure-to-come infirmities. The cold winter air hurt my chest, and I'd have to wrap my long woolen scarf around my face to breathe in warmed air. Sure enough, I'd catch a cold and be whisked off to the doctor for more exams and antibiotics. Sinus infections were frequent in this proverbial "blockhead". Nasal sprays worked for a few minutes, but that remedy would soon backfire, closing them tighter than before (rebound effect). Migraine headaches plagued me and lasted sometimes for two weeks at a clip. Ear Nose and Throat specialists offered to remove the sinuses to cure my problem. In my early twenties, painfully swollen fingers and toes were diagnosed as poly-inflammatory arthritis. The rheumatologist put me on a course of fourteen aspirin a day for several weeks. The inflammation did subside, along with my digestion. Several more specialists for other health problems basically gave "pats on the back", prescriptions and encouraging words to "keep doing what you're doing."

Hello? It's Not Working!

In my mid-thirties the birth of two beautiful children brought us faithfully to pediatricians. On these many visits, I was noticing more and more that diagnoses and resulting treatments were dubious at best. It was routine to give my daughter Tylenol whenever she had an injection to be sure to keep an expected fever down. Once, the doctor prescribed antibiotics for her slightly pink ear just in case an infection developed. The final straw came when I took my daughter, now two, in for a cough-laced chest cold. "She has asthma.", the doctor announced. He told me emphatically that she needed to be started on a drug called Ventalin.

"Ventalin?" I asked. "Yes", he responded, "it is a narcotic and the medicine of choice in these cases."

I was becoming quite upset at what I was hearing-- at both the diagnosis and the proposed treatment. A two year old on a narcotic? She had no symptoms before. No-- there must be something else. The more I persisted in my questions and protests, the more adamant the doctor became. He reminded me that I knew nothing and he knew everything.

"No, I do not want to give her Ventalin," I insisted. "What other options do we have?"

I will never forget his words, as the anger flared and his neck and face reddened.

"Who do you think you are questioning my expertise. I am the doctor!"

Becoming very annoyed at his impatience and haughtiness, I responded, "Yes, well, I'm her mother, responsible for her life, and you won't be seeing us again!"

All the way home I reflected upon that disagreeable visit, angry and yet scared. Once in the house, I put the children to bed for a nap and started down the stairs to the kitchen. The wheels started turning again on this whole unhealthy business-- sick to well, sick to well, and sick again, all too often. And, how about myself? My weight was climbing and my energy spent, like only one prong was in the outlet. I fancied myself a very disciplined person, but not where my cravings for sweets were concerned. Homemade cherry pies were my nemesis. At least three times a week, I'd roll out the dough made from white flour to make two pie crusts. Salivating like a boxer pup, I'd open two cans of pie cherries. Those bright red, round little fruits in the sugary red syrup would have to be sampled, at least several tablespoonfuls before dumping the rest in the pie shells. The diligent baker would open the oven many times to smell the aroma and check for a nice golden hue. The knife and spatula were well in hand before one pie would be completely cooled to section it off for "tastes". One down, and one to go-- for after dinner. "Yes, dear. I'll have one dainty slice or maybe two."

At the bottom, Looking Up

Something was terribly wrong, and my efforts were not working. I began to cry my eyes out. Desperate for change, I prayed with all my might. I asked God to please give me direction on how to get well. To be fruitful, productive, energetic, raising a healthy family and helping others was not too big a request. Feeling sure my answer would come, I sat quietly, hopeful. It came not quite an hour later.

The telephone rang, and a friend of mine asked me to attend a lecture at a local health food store and take notes for her. She was going out of town and didn't want to miss it. My mind started racing: "I go to M.D.s, and I worked in the medical field ten years. Wasn't this health food stuff just quackery? Those people eat birdseed, cardboard and bicycle seats like Uhl Gibbons. I guess that little gourmet grocery store in Phoenix with the gingham curtains and country-fied decor, with lots of oak and wooden floors, was somewhat like a health food store."

"Sue, are you there? Are you listening?"

"Oh, sorry Ann. I was just thinking."

Ready to decline her request, I remembered my fervent prayer. Maybe this was my answer, so sheepishly the assignment was accepted.

Ann told me the topic to be discussed was candida albicans. That sounded to me like a rare species of birds. Actually, I learned it was "yeasts" not "beasts".

Sure enough, going to that lecture changed my life. It was common sense, logic and intelligent reason offered by Ria Gilday, a knowledgeable and highly-qualified nutritionist. At the conclusion, I scheduled an appointment to meet with her. When the time arrived, she wanted to know why I came. There were many health reasons, but I blurted out, "to lose weight." Her response surprised and intrigued me. She said, "If you want to lose weight, exercise and choose from a number of safe, natural products. But, if you want to learn how to take care of yourself and get well, we'll talk." Yes! Taking care of myself and getting well was why I came, and I immediately saw that commitment to healthy changes would be what it would take. Over the course of a year, my health and the health of my children improved remarkably. It took dedication, determination and responsibility for what I was learning. Many doctors told me I would have to live with allergies, arthritis, chronic fatigue and without my sinuses. I'm happy to tell you I don't for almost twenty years. My daughter never took that narcotic, nor does she have asthma. I am so thankful both children have good health from wholesome living. With deep gratitude and eagerness, I've pursued further education for an expanded life's work. My prayer has been answered abundantly, assisting many clients on the road to vibrant health by teaching them healthy living habits.

What It Takes

Daily we are faced with choices that will impact our health positively or negatively. Whether it is what we are thinking and dwelling upon, what we are putting in and on our bodies, or what is present in our environment, the cause is there to contribute to or take away from our overall health. If we eat, drink, wear, inhale or think unhealthy, damaging things, what can we expect? You know GIGO-- garbage in, garbage out. Toxemia, in all its forms, is the primary cause of disease. We'll discuss this much more in upcoming chapters.

Good health is about changes, about growth and living to have a renewed, refreshed body and spirit. Learn to recognize what tears us down physically, emotionally and spiritually. Cultivate a willingness to new perceptions, enlightenment offering effective results. Upcoming chapters examine how and why we should eat the right foods, prepare them for maximum nutritional benefit, exercise properly and regularly, take in enough fresh air and sunshine, feed the spirit, reject harmful thoughts, meet the demands of stress and get adequate rest. We'll look at these precepts in a more detailed way to encourage you if you're skeptical or curious to know what a natural approach to wellness entails. If you're already living a healthy lifestyle, I hope it encourages you to continue and to enthusiastically spread the word with every opportunity. You may also find this a fitting gift for someone you love who doesn't know where to start.

Let us demand of our health care professionals to teach us how to live correctly and not just manage disease. Alternative caregivers have been doing that for decades in this country and centuries in others. Our students are taught that daily habits create the environment for health or disease. By identifying and removing the disease-causing conditions in our life, we will be on the side of true prevention.

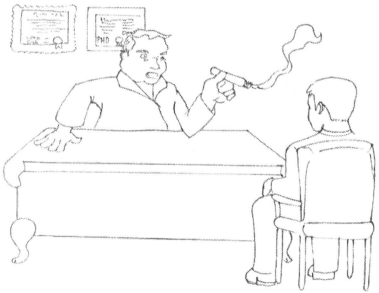

"I'M PUTTING YOU ON A DIET FOR YOUR HEALTH."

CHAPTER TWO

CLOSE-UP ON HEALTH

Man cannot discover
new oceans until he has
courage to lose sight of the shore.

Unknown

A Mental Picture

Take a moment to close your eyes while you picture a vibrant, healthy person. And now, describe in detail what you see. (Go ahead, close your eyes.)

Did you see thick, shiny hair, clear sparkling eyes with whites really white, framed with long, dark lashes, rosy cheeks on a creamy, glowing skin, a fit, toned, muscular body slightly tanned, and highly-energized, ready for work or play, with a ready, radiant smile? Your description of this fantasy person could be you! Hippocrates, known as the Father of Medicine, said, "A wise man should consider that health is the greatest of human blessings."

Health is defined as the general condition of the body or mind; soundness of body or mind; freedom from disease or ailment, vigor; vitality. (1)

---

(1) The Oxford American Desk Dictionary, 2001

Health is built from cellular level on up. More than one hundred different kinds of cells have been identified in the human body, and they are all programmed to perform specific functions. Each individual cell can be likened to an infinitely small, walled-in city. Genetics or heredity factors is the government, maintaining law and order. Power plants within generate energy, and manufacturing plants produce proteins. These chemical commodities are carried to locations within and beyond the city by complex transportation systems. Guards posted at the entrances oppose outside threats while monitoring and controlling incoming and outgoing goods. When foreign invaders attack, they are met by a highly-skilled and disciplined army equipped in biological warfare.

Cells join together to form tissues; two or more tissues grouped together form structural and functional units called organs. A group of organs functions harmoniously to carry out principal activities of the body, and we call these organ systems. Specialized cells which produce and discharge substances are called glands. Our organ systems, made up of molecules, cells, tissues, and organs, interact with one another keep us alive and well. This state of "wellness" when everything is doing its programmed job individually and jointly is called homeostasis. Homeostasis, therefore, is the maintenance of a stable or balanced internal environment despite what may be a very different external one. Given the right conditions, right fuel, and a balanced approach to living, we can maintain good internal balance. We lose this balance due to a variety of reasons, but two bottom-line reasons would be toxemia and malnutrition.

Here A Symptom, There a Symptom

If the imbalance continues, we start to manifest symptoms. To illustrate, human blood normally should have a higher calcium to phosphorus ratio. When a person drinks too many soft drinks which are high in phosphorus, the calcium/phosphorus ratios become reversed. The body is signaled to draw upon the calcium stored in bones to normalize these undesirable blood levels. Pulling upon the bone stores of calcium like this over a period of time without correcting the deficit can lead to aching joints, slow pulse, leg cramps, muscle tics and twitches, loose teeth, nervousness, and irritability-- all symptoms. Eventually, osteoporosis may result. Chronic conditions such as arthritis, heart disease, diabetes and cancer still plague us although there has been intense scientific research and astounding advancements in medical technology. High-tech equipment, sophisticated lab tests, and designer drugs seem to hold promise of great success during periods of remissions. However, when deterioration proceeds with worsening symptoms, all the prevention measures and professed cures alike are purely academic. It's back to the drawing board, anticipating millions of dollars in grants and donations to discover yet again a new cure.

One wonders, when will the microscope magnify and illuminate the causes of disease? We may not want to admit it, but the modern tools of medicine are often of themselves more invasive and radical, causing serious side effects. Chemotherapy and radiation are certainly two such examples. There are others less well known to cause problems but they are insidious nonetheless. Consider simple over the counter medications that are taken without any concern. . Ibuprofen, a common pain reliever: possible side effects of dizziness, drowsiness, headache, mild abdominal pain, constipation or diarrhea, heartburn or nausea, anaphylactic reaction, gastrointestinal bleeding, ulceration, stomach perforation, angina, diminished hearing or ringing in the ears, fluid retention, jaundice or blood in the urine. (2) You can check these facts in The Physicians Desk Reference or PDR which lists all prescription and non-prescription drugs along with their use, contraindications and side effects.

In cases of trauma, injuries and other life-threatening emergencies, heroes trained in modern medicine rise to the call, and precious lives are saved that might otherwise have been lost. But, when it comes to chronic health problems or what is commonly called "disease", western medicine has lagged behind. The real emphasis and success of alternative health care has always been to prevent illness in the first place. These approaches are generally less expensive, very effective and safer when addressing everyday health issues. They also offer far more than palliative measures. The changes are deeper, addressing the underlying causes of the symptoms. We strive to create an environment where disease cannot gain a foothold.

Let us digress once more to this matter of synthetic drugs. Some drugs banish or reduce debilitating symptoms. The watchword here is

(2) The Drug and Natural Medicine Advisor c 1997, Time Life Books

"symptom". A symptom is an alarm going off-- something is wrong. It is your smoke detector. What is more annoying than a smoke detector doing its job? It alerts you to a low battery or perhaps there is smoke and fire! You don't disconnect it without checking for the cause. This is an important correlation with the human body. It nudges us, then nags us and finally screams at us so loudly we do something major to stop it. In case the smoke detector example didn't impress enough, let's look at it another way... treating the symptom is like mopping up the bathroom floor because the tub is overflowing. Slight progress is being made in the cleanup since no one's bothered to turn off the faucet. You can use sponge mops, string mops, buckets and even wet vacs for a month of Sundays-- but the cleanup will keep going on until someone decides to look for the tap and shut it off or you can no longer breathe under water.

Headaches, coughs, stomach aches, sneezing, fevers, diarrhea, muscle and joint aches, swelling, rashes, depression, blurred vision, and all the rest are symptoms. We opt for symptomatic relief and begin a viscious cycle of "here a symptom, there a pill, here another symptom, there another pill." Each new side-effect has a companion pill to alleviate it.

I've spoken to countless people who take antacids for heartburn. A convenient swallow and the fire is out! However, now that the antacid has cooled the symptom, digestive capacity is reduced, and the stomach acid needed for digestion is neutralized. The food at this point is not going to be broken down to the degree necessary to pass into the small intestine, and the result will be gas, bloating and intestinal discomfort. There may also be constipation. So, now an over-the-counter laxative is chosen which pulls water, minerals and other important nutrients from the intestines, weakening the peristaltic action with frequent use. Prolonged use of antacids and laxatives may cause a dangerous imbalance in minerals. Aggravating symptoms often keep one awake, so a pain pill and sleep-aid are taken. In the morning, there is fatigue and the feeling of being "drugged." It might take a few extra cups of caffeine to wake up. Do you see domino effect that results from not addressing the cause of the very first problem-- heartburn? Pill-popping is an answer, but does it make sense? What is causing the heartburn may be a poor diet with excessive consumption of spicy, fried and fatty foods, or combining foods poorly, ulcers, gallbladder problems, allergies, enzyme deficiency, stress or perhaps too much or too little hydrochloric acid in the stomach. The Big Question: Why is it so hard to ask ourselves what we are not doing right? And then and make some changes? When the cause is removed, no more symptoms. Our bodies respond really well to intelligent, supportive therapies. Whether we face serious health issues or merely have a few bad habits, we can proceed a step at a time to address our total needs. Health will result when you live it.

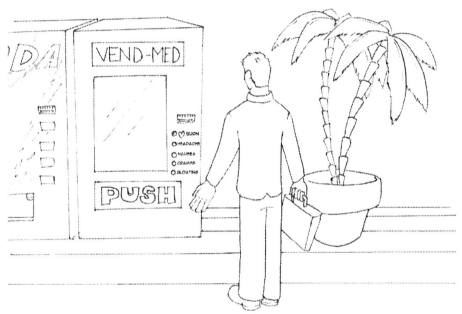

"LETS SEE. IF I GET NUMBER ONE I'M GONNA NEED ALL FIVE."

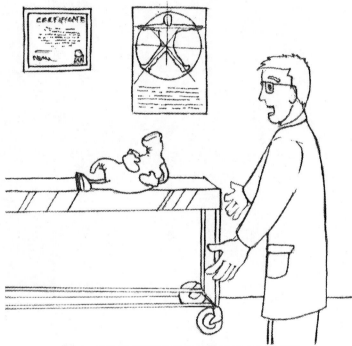

"I'LL GIVE YOU SOMETHING FOR
A STOMACHACHE."

CHAPTER THREE

INTRODUCING A BIOCHEMICALLY UNIQUE 'YOU'

A million snowflakes, a dozen roses,
each unique in beauty all its own.
A brilliant diamond, a flashy emerald
sparkling brightly unlike any precious stone.
Of all the people who have lived
and those who are to come,
there won't be another just like you.
Yes, you're uniquely one.

"Reflecting on Life," Susanne

Yesterday and Today

Snowflakes, fingerprints and you-- no two exactly alike. There has never been nor ever will there be anyone totally like you, cloning aside. That biological uniqueness is very important to consider when you want to begin a program of wellness.

Our parents pass on their genes to us with their strengths and weaknesses. Because of that we have pre-dispositions to various health issues. We also see conditions which "run" in families due to lifestyle similarities. The future need not be gloomy and the inherent weaknesses so glaringly apparent if the body is given the needed support and correct conditions to counteract these realities.

George Burns lived to be over 100 despite plentiful cigars and alcohol. Indeed, some individuals can abuse themselves more than others and still live longer. We good-naturedly chalk it up to "good genes." People in other civilizations and cultures live to be 120, even over 150 because it is genetically possible.

Our forefathers farmed the land and ate largely from their own gardens--- wholesome food without additives and preservatives. They did not eat highly-processed junk foods. They also didn't run to the doctor's office every month for the latest designer drug. I recall my Mom telling me how she and her brother, Leo, were playing cowboys and Indians when he sank a hatchet into her scalp-- a real, honest-to-goodness hatchet. She ran into the house, crying and bleeding. Uncle Leo followed closely behind crying and apologetic. Nana called Dr. Pavaledis, the town doctor, who promptly walked to their house, neither horse and buggy nor a Mercedes for him! He poured medicine into the cut and put a bandage on it. The kids went back out to play leaving the hatchet indoors. There were no ER forms, health cards, or x-rays. No tetanus shot was given and there was no waiting "forever" in a lobby while onlookers stare at your problem. My mom also remembers one-week stays in the hospital for giving birth to two children at a total cost of $48.00 for the first, $52.00 for the second. Not quite the inflationary figures of today.

In many cases, the doctor wasn't available at all, and you did the best you could. Nana went outside and noticed one of her pet ducks was flailing and flopping around in distress. She caught him and determined he had swallowed a locust which got stuck in his neck. After yelling for her neighbor, Mrs. Schwartz, to hold the duck still, Nana did a "tracheotomy" and removed the locust. She took needle and thread, closed the incision and off he went, none worse for the wear.

We know how different today's world is, how much more complex it is, with environmental concerns and dangers ever present. My great grandfather, Ed Freeman, was a sheriff in Afton, Oklahoma. My grandfather, Hugh, was a crane operator, and my father, Bert, worked as a millwright, carpenter and welder. Dad worked on commercial buildings and also on nuclear plants-- certainly, a very different world from that of his father and grandfather.

As each successive generation has come on the scene, we see the effects of a lifestyle becoming more and more unnatural. Look at our youth today. Instead of chronic health problems such as arthritis, diabetes, and obesity occurring at ages forty and fifty, we see it now in teens as well as twenty and thirty year olds. These problems are largely the result of the foods we eat and nutritional deficiencies that are not being addressed. We're feeding our kids food grown in over-farmed, nutrient-depleted soils, food that is over-processed, devitalized, irradiated, preserved, genetically modified, dyed, nuked and artificially flavored. We're putting real lemons in furniture polish, while artificial lemon flavors their sugary drinks. We encourage them, bribe them and reward them with sugar.

"Just a spoonful helps the medicine go down."

"If you clear your plate, you can have an ice cream sundae."

"If you behave at the store, I will buy you a treat."

And let's not forget the absolutely absurd, unhealthy products that are marketed to youth. While standing in a checkout line in a department store, my son noticed a display. "Hey, check this out! Look at this can of spray paint for your hair." It was a Halloween special of iridescent paint in bright, bold colors. As my kids became interested in which of those colors were their favorites, I turned the can to expose the WARNING LABEL. "Contents extremely toxic. Purposely inhaling fumes may cause death." This--- on a product specifically sold to spray on your head! What a great impulse item to have in the check-out line for the kids to buy. My son and daughter, saucer-eyed, quickly lost interest.

Too Many Toxins

Is it any wonder we have aches and pains and feel lousy? Not only are our children unaware of what is unhealthy, even dangerous, adults are sadly in the dark as well. I had a client, Betty, whom I met in a department store in Albuquerque, who was diagnosed by her doctor as having multiple sclerosis. She was experiencing headaches, joint aches, difficulty with concentration and walking, and she was so afraid of the progression of her condition. Hopeful that something "natural" might help, Betty asked me to assist her. Upon investigating her lifestyle, it was evident she was exposed to a plethora of toxins everyday. At work, she opened and emptied many boxes of new clothing. The garments and plastic wrappings out-gassed toxic fumes from dyes, formaldehyde and other hazardous ingredients. The woolen suits she wore to work every day were laden with chemicals through the dry-cleaning process. The bugs outside her front door were a constant problem, and for them she sprayed insecticides almost every evening to keep them away. She took various medications for breathing problems, sinus infections, and headaches and was on a frequent round of antibiotics. A friend she saw often for social drinking occasions was a heavy smoker. After her eyes were opened to all the toxic exposures she was receiving, a whole new vista of health appreciation unfolded for her. Betty was determined to clean up her environment, both internally and externally, and once she took action to reduce her toxic intake, she saw marked improvement in her health.

Smoke, The Missing Clue

The cause of toxicity problems is not always obvious. My Dad was always strong like a bull with a healthy physique from hard work and good clean living. More than ten years ago on a hot summer day, he was raking leaves and clearing brush in the field near a pond. He had a rare cold, and his sense of smell was not acute. All of a sudden, his legs gave out and he fell to the ground, feeling quite dizzy. When he was able to collect himself, he made it up to the house some distance away, sank into a kitchen chair, looking pale. Mom and Dad discussed what happened. They decided that he had become overcome with heat, and had perhaps sustained sunstroke. As the next few days progressed, Dad had more symptoms of dizziness, his gait was off, his right arm and hand became numb, his speech slurred and soon his mouth twisted on the right side. The family doctor referred him to a neurologist for tests. Everyone suspected a stroke. All the tests came back negative. Several more days passed and his condition worsened. It seemed that paralysis was setting in and would be permanent. What was going on? While the tests were negative, something still, very obviously, was seriously wrong.

The property adjoining my parents belongs to a commercial business. An employee of this company had gone behind the building and, totally unaware of any danger, began to burn empty plastic containers which held muriatic acid and chlorine. This toxic smoke had drifted down to where Dad was working. Once he remembered being in smoke shortly before his legs gave out, we were able to understand that an extreme toxic insult was disabling his health. Someone with a lesser build, not as strong and healthy, may not have survived. A rigorous program was begun to cleanse his system and rebuild it with therapeutic amounts of important nutrients. It took almost a year for his body to recover from that assault.

Red Hot Mounds

Connie was a woman in her early thirties who approached me very distraught about her health. Her doctor was sure she had lupus and had referred her to a specialist. She was awaiting definitive testing, but in the meantime she wanted to see what could be done nutritionally to build herself up. For two weeks, she had been experiencing extreme joint pain; she proceeded to show me both her wrists. On the lateral side (outside) of each wrist were what looked like miniature volcano-shaped mounds, red and hot to the touch. I was curious to know if she could remember anything in her life or routine preceding this past two-week time period that was different in this time period. She couldn't think of a thing.

"What type of work do you do?" I asked.

"I clean houses for a living.", she responded.

"Have you bought anything new to use on the job?"

"No", she replied unable to recall anything unusual.

As we talked, I still had suspicions of a recent toxic exposure.

"Are you sure nothing unusual happened with chemicals or products you might have used?", I persisted.

Her faced turned white, as she suddenly remembered something. It was an incident when she had accidentally mixed Clorox with ammonia on one of her cleaning jobs. She remembered breathing the vapors and passing out briefly. The "mounds" appeared several days afterwards. Clorox and ammonia can be a deadly combination. We worked on cleansing as well as supporting the immune system, (3) and within about ten days her wrists were back to normal and the joints improved considerably.

Why Are We Missing the Cause?

It is not surprising that environmental factors affecting health go unnoticed. Two very important facts are reported by the Chemical Injury Information Network based in Montana:

❖ Only 2% of the doctors in the United States are qualified to diagnose chemical poisoning and its related problems. (4) And,

❖ No toxicity data is available for the 80% of some 49,000 chemicals in commercial use. Of the more than 70,000 chemicals in daily use, complete toxicity data is available on only 2%. (5)

(3) Cleansing: plenty of pure water, fresh vegetable juices, herbs and superfoods and gentle natural bulking agents for the colon; also, antioxidants for immune support.

(4) Institute of Medicine, Division of Health Promotion & Disease Prevention, Role of the Primary Care Physician in Occupational and Environmental Medicine (1988), National Academy Press

(5) US Congress, Neurotoxicity: Identifying and Controlling Poisons of the Nervous System, Office of Technology Assessment, April, 1990, US Government Printing Office, Washington, DC and US Congress, "Neurotoxins: At Home and the Workplace," 99th Congress, 2nd Session, April 24, 1987, Senate Hearing 100-70, printed for use of the Committee on Environment & Public Works, US Government Printing Office, Washington, DC

A Sick Sentence

When Sharon walked into my office, she came in all slumped over with the weight of the world on her shoulders. I could see immediately she was depressed, without any light of hope or joy in her eyes. She had been diagnosed with asthma, a spastic colon, severe depression, agoraphobia, and other health problems. She felt that her life was a waste, without purpose, and she figured she might as well be dead. Her doctor did not mince words stating that she should be institutionalized for her depression. He painted the bleakest of pictures, telling her she would never be well again.

Those words raised a fury in me, and I couldn't help but retort on Sharon's first visit, "Oh, and he is God?" She raised her head, and for the first time looked me straight in the eye. Sharon actually smiled, and gave out a short giggle. Then she resumed her former posture, dejection overtaking her.

"I'm sorry, I continued, " if you want to buy into that sentence, you go right ahead. I personally believe we do have choices in these matters."

Sharon and I began, slowly at first, to investigate those choices. We identified lifestyle changes needing to be made in order to have a healthier body, clear mind and strong spirit.

It took a number of months, but with each passing month, I began to see a lovely, industrious, vital woman emerging. (6)

To assess one's health needs, you and your health professional must consider all aspects of your past and present lifestyle to ascertain where there may be apparent nutritional deficiencies, imbalances and toxic exposures. This exercise probably will require some serious mental work, as you consider all the aspects about the way you have lived. But if you do your homework, you'll be much more helpful to your health practitioner. You can begin by spending some time with the following Health Assessment Questionnaire exercise:

---

(6) It was necessary to make major dietary changes, use supplements therapeutically, address colon health, incorporate an exercise regimen and cultivate a more positive outlook.

1)   What did I eat growing up? What foods do I now crave?

2)   What percentage of my food do I eat raw and what percentage is cooked? How is my food prepared?

3)   What type of cooking utensils were used growing up and at present?

4)   What major periods of stress have I gone through? How have I coped with this stress?

5)   What over the counter medications have I taken for any length of time? (Aspirin, antacids, cough medicine, etc.)

6)   What prescription drugs have I taken over the years?

7)   What occupations have I had? Were they sedentary jobs? Did they   expose me to any environmental toxins, chemicals, etc.?

8)   What are my sleep habits?

9)   Have I used any illegal substances like marijuana, cocaine, heroin,etc.?

10) Have I abused alcohol for any period of time? How often do I drink alcohol?

11) What childhood diseases did I have? What immunizations did I have?

12) What health conditions are prevalent in my immediate family? (father, mother, brothers, sisters)

13) What health challenges am I presently encountering?

14) What surgeries have I had?

15) Have I used any chemicals or toxic products at work, recreation, home or for hobbies?

16) Have I had pets over the years which may have exposed me to parasites? (Cats, dogs and horses, for example, harbor many different types of parasites transmittable to humans.)

17) Have I traveled abroad or eaten raw meats or fish? Have I had any bouts with intestinal flu, vomiting or diarrhea shortly after a trip abroad?

18) Do I routinely drink tap water?

19) Soft drinks? Coffee? Tea? How often and how much?

20) Do I used artificial sweetners?

21) What are my exercise habits?

22)   Have I had root canals or major dental work?

23)   How often have I taken antibiotics?

24)   What are my bowel habits?

25)   Do I now use or have I in the past used tobacco? Explain.

26)   Is my system alkaline or acidic?

27)   How is my outlook and general disposition?

28)   What are my health goals, prioritized?

This partial list considers some of the major aspects of our physicality. Delving into these and along with other questions about physical, mental, emotional and spiritual health will help you and your health practitioners appreciate how unique you are and help you understand why you are in your present state of health. A thorough understanding of where we've been, where we are now and where we want to be will bring about an appropriate, effective program.

CHAPTER FOUR

WHERE IS OUR FOOD GETTING US?

Trusting so-called authority is not enough. A sense of personal responsibility is what we desperately need.

Rachel Carson, Biologist and Gifted Nature Writer

Food, Glorious Food

Eating is one of life's most pleasurable experiences. You could say we have a love affair with food. We share joys, important events, meet new friends, court each other, solve problems and make business deals over food. "Let's do lunch." As a matter of fact, the majestic pineapple is a symbol for hospitality, showing how closely connected the serving of food is with being hospitable.

We look forward to the gathering of friends and family at mealtimes to share the high points of the day. Each place setting at the table is beautifully arranged with brightly-colored place mats and napkins. The napkin rings are an unusual and artful complement. Freshly cut buttercups, cornflowers, day lilies and daises add a palette of brilliant matching colors and gently scent the air. In the background, soft music creates a relaxing mood. From the kitchen comes the aroma of fresh herbs, spices, garlic, and onions. Something wonderful is sautéing on the stove while fresh baked, whole grain sourdough bread cools on a rack nearby. A huge tray of creatively arranged fresh vegetables is served alongside bowls of assorted homemade dips-- hummus, tomato-avocado, and bean with green chilies. In high spirits, everyone comes to the table ready to experience all the skillfully prepared, mouthwatering dishes from our carefully-tended organic garden. (Wait-- is this too idyllic?) OK-- we sit down together to a hot TV dinner, pop a roll in the toaster oven and tell each other what a rough day we've had. (Still not there?) We stop at the closest drive-thrus on the way home, gulping down fast foods and ice-cold soft drinks, then we're off to our separate activities. Kids are rushed to their appointments or friends houses, and us to our meetings. "Hi!" "Bye!"

Food and Health

Food is one of the most important facets of health. I feel it is the foundation. It contains nutrients-- vitamins, minerals, enzymes, amino acids, fats, water and hydrocarbons. These nutrients supply the basic materials our bodies need to function every day. That old adage, You are what you eat" is true along with what you digest, absorb and assimilate. This is why so many Americans are in trouble. We eat the wrong things at a frantic pace. We perpetually snack since we're not getting the minerals and other nutrients we need from our food. Daily, the average American consumes 4,000 to 6,000 mg. of sodium. In a year's time, the average American consumes about 165 pounds of sugar and in a lifetime, about a half ton of assorted animals. These animals have been pumped up with antibiotics, growth hormones, pesticide-laden feed, and are raised in overcrowded pens without the ability to roam and graze. Once slaughtered, the meat is treated with additives and preservatives.

I recently saw a program on the importing of beef from Mexico. As the animals crossed the border, they were counted and herded into corrals where inspectors would try to ascertain any sick animals. Those with respiratory problems were marked. The rest were then sent through a chute to jump into a rectangular pool of neck deep pesticide/insecticide. Yummy! Anyone for a nice "juicy" steak? Can we also fathom herbivorous (vegetarian) cattle being fed feed made from animal carcasses, including cows and sheep infected with scrapie? This practice is exactly what has been done, and researchers conclude that mad cow disease (bovine spongiform encephalopathy) in humans is in all probability attributed to eating BSE infected meat.

Oh, no! It's a GMO!

Whole, unprocessed foods were eaten by our ancestors for generations, but science came along and enlightened businesses on how to take shortcuts for profits with the food chain. Crops were now sprayed with poisonous, cancer-causing pesticides, foods can stay on shelves for a year or more, and now, we have fish genes combining with tomatoes. The fish/tomato comment, of course, refers to the technology of genetically-modified organisms or GMOs. This technology of genetically- modified food focuses on manipulating the DNA inside the cells of living things to block or add desired traits.

NATURAL FOODS MERCHANDISER, a trade magazine for the natural foods industry, has been tracking the GMO news reports and keeping us posted on the latest developments. Here are highlights from some recent articles:

❖ In the September 2000, issue an article entitled "Health Threat Looms Over GMO Debate" reported GMO genes in food crops can jump from one species to another and can cause bacteria to mutate, according to a zoologist working in Germany. After a four-year study, "Professor Kaatz of the Institute for Bee Research at the University of Jena found that genes used to modify oilseed rape (canola) were transferred to bacteria in the guts of bees. He experimented with honey bees and GM oilseed rape, which has been modified to resist a specific herbicide." He removed the pollen from the legs of bees and fed it to young bees. When he examined the young bees' intestines, he found that some carried the gene that resisted the herbicide. Scientists are concerned about genetic traits jumping species because "one of the genes used in genetic engineering by agricultural sciences companies is a gene resistant to antibiotics used as a marker-- something like a genetic sticker on fruit that can't be removed." The article quoted Joe Cummins, Ph.D.., professor emeritus of genetics at the University of Western Ontario, Canada, who stated, "The spread of antibiotic resistance is the main threat from gene transfer from GM crops." "I have found that the antibiotics used in GM crops are used in surgery to treat a number of diseases."

❖ In October, 2000, issue an article appeared by Scott Yates entitled, "Monsanto's PR Money Isn't Buying The GMO Leader a Break."

He stated, "In a repeat of news that sparked the biggest public interest in genetically modified organisms so far in the United States, a published study has shown that corn modified to kill harmful pests also kills monarch butterfly larvae. The study performed by Iowa State University and published in the journal Oecologia showed that half of the monarch larvae died within three days of exposure to pollen from genetically modified corn. None of the larvae exposed to non-GMO pollen died. Yates also stated, "One of the researchers said the study shows that not enough research was done before the US government approved the corn.... After a report from Cornell University last year, the monarch became the most visible symbol of those fighting GMOs."

❖ The November, 2001, issue under "GE Update: Biotech.com Invades Mexico: "Mexico's Ministry of the Environment and Natural Resources announced in September that as much as 10% of corn seed tested in 22 communities in the state of Oaxaca have been contaminated with genetically engineered DNA of Bt corn. Regulators haven't determined the full extent of the contamination, and efforts to quantify the problem are hindered because they don't know exactly how it happened. Two years ago, Mexico forbade the cultivation of biotech corn, which has been grown in the United States since 1996." A microbial ecologist at University of California stated, "The only reason they found it there is because that's the only place they've looked." Also in the same article, "The findings are worrisome. From Oaxaca to Chihuahua, there is amazing diversity of maize plants, as well as a wild relative called teosinte. Both are likely threatened as the biotech corn is engineered with an advantageous trait that allows the plant to produce its own pesticide".

The same article further announced that "rice fields in the Sacramento Valley, not far from thousands of acres of farmland under organic cultivation, are planted by pharmaceutical researchers with a trial crop of GM rice engineered with *human* genes." These crops are being grown as potential drugs and not meant for human consumption. Although Applied Phytologics, Inc., a research and development firm with ties to the University of California at Davis, said it has taken the necessary precautions so as not to affect surrounding fields, environmental and organic advocates fear the worst. "Greenpeace Science Adviser Doreen Stabinsky pointed out that the Central Valley is one stop on the migration trail for millions of ducks. Those ducks eat leftover rice in fields, and rice seed sowed by air will grow where the ducks drop it."

❖ From May, 2002, issue, it was reported that "a recently released study from the European Environment Agency confirmed the worst fears of environmentalists and members of the organic industry. Transgenic genes will inevitably escape from genetically modified crops, contaminating organic farms, creating superweeds and driving wild plants to extinction."

With such implications, we should all be concerned about the impact of GMOs on the environment. This technology has been applied to crops, processed foods and dairy products from cows injected with recombinant bovine growth hormone. There are no laws mandating that ingredients must be labeled as genetically modified, so you may be consuming them whether you want to or not. If this concerns you, you can e-mail from the TAKE ACTION NOW section of the Center for Food Safety's web site: www.centerforfoodsafety.org. You can also write or call your Senator and Congressperson to let them know you support mandatory labeling and food safety bills. We can all support manufacturers making a difference by providing non-genetically modified ingredients within their products.

Irradiation

Foods are also being irradiated. Irradiation is a method of killing insects and bacteria as well as preserving by treating with low doses of gamma radiation from Cobalt 60 or the radioactive isotope Cesium 137, a byproduct of nuclear weapon production and nuclear power plants. Although the food is not radioactive per se, the chemical structure is altered. Nutrients are destroyed and untested compounds are created called URPs (unique radiolytic products). Many of these are feared to be potent carcinogens. Supporters for irradiation, especially public health and government officials, have begun a campaign to promote increased use of irradiation to decrease the risk of food borne illness. It sounds to me like shouting the praises for the lesser of two evils. There needs to be an acute emphasis on sanitation and safe food handling practices in the whole process of getting foods to market. However, as long as that rush to market is driven solely by the profit motive, it doesn't allow for the sane and safe way to do things. Our Standard American Diet (SAD) has never been more adulterated and nutritionally deficient. History does seem to repeat itself. We have reaped the lack of foresight in many a new technology that was going to bring "better life through chemistry."

Pasteurization and Homogenization

Pasteurization was a good idea before the advent of refrigeration and proper sterilization techniques. It served to benefit the farmers the expense of proper sanitary conditions in large-scale, mechanized production plants. It calls for integrity, care and conscientiousness to be sure the animal and equipment are "pristine" clean. As it stands, a certain percentage of E. coli is allowed by the government to show up in the bottled milk. Perhaps this is why it turns sour when the date is still good. Nutrient-wise, pasteurization reduces vitamins such as B6 by 50%. Homogenization takes the globules of fat from the cream which settles on top of the milk and breaks them apart to a more uniform size. These molecules of fat are then absorbed by our small intestines, heightening the risk of allergies and atherosclerosis. In other countries, cheese ages over a period of time. But, here in America, it can be done in a few hours or days.

Hydrogenation

Hydrogenation infuses hydrogen into poly-unsaturated oil to reconstruct its chemical bonds and slow down rancidity. Rancid oils are very toxic to the system causing serious health problems. This process transforms a liquid such as corn oil into a solid-- margarine. The body is unable to use this now "saturated fat" which is solid at room temperature. I've heard many a respectable nutritionist liken margarine to axle grease. Hydrogenation creates unhealthy trans-fatty acids. They can cause platelet aggregation which is a clumping or sticking together of blood platelets. This increases the likelihood of blood clots in small vessels. They may be combined with aluminum or nickel used as a catalyst in processing; both heavy metals are toxic to us in cumulative amounts. They can decrease the performance of the heart muscle. Be aware that oils are refined to the point of being almost nutrient-free just like white flour and sugar. They are degummed to keep them from going rancid, removing vitamin E. They are de-pigmented, clarified, deodorized under high heat and chemically preserved. Solvents like hexane, a petroleum based chemical, are used for maximum extraction. A healthier alternative to margarine and shortening would be to combine equal parts of a cold-pressed, virgin vegetable oil with equal parts of organic butter. Blend or mix with hand mixer and store in a closed glass container in the refrigerator. You may include a pierced capsule or two of vitamin E as a preservative.

Fats

There is still among dieters the fat-free, low-fat and no-fat frenzy. As in the case with much information disseminated to the public, it becomes oversimplified, misleading or just plain erroneous due to the profit motive. There have been more than enough books published within the past few years to squelch this misconception of fats. We need to know there are good fats in white hats and bad fats in black hats. Fatty acids are building blocks of all oils and fats, both in foods and in our bodies. They are a primary ingredient in our cell membranes and are vital to the construction and maintenance of all healthy cells. Trans-fatty acids are the bad guys for the reasons already mentioned. Saturated fats are those from meat or butter. Eating too much of these can clog arteries and lead to degenerative problems. But here the emphasis is on too much. Unsaturated fats are also known as mono or poly-unsaturated fats from vegetation or nuts, and these are liquid at room temperature. These are the major source for essential fatty acids-- linoleic, linolenic and arachidonic-- required for our bodies for proper cell membrane function, balancing prostaglandins and other metabolic processes. (Prostaglandins are a vital group of hormone-like substances that result from essential fatty acids and regulate body functions electrically.) Ocean fish, sea foods, sunflower, safflower and olive oils, evening primrose oil, borage oil and flax oil all affect the prostaglandin balance. Poly-unsaturated oils help reduce serum cholesterol provided adequate dietary fiber is present. Buy cold-pressed, unrefined or virgin oils and organic butter, and remember to store them in the refrigerator. Cold-pressed means no heat is used to extract the oil, and it is used primarily with olive oil.

Essential fatty acids cannot be made by the body and must be supplied through the diet. Eating bad fats interferes with the proper utilization of essential fatty acids which are important for brain function, nerve health, hormone development, reproduction and fertility, immunity, preventing hardening of the arteries, reducing the growth rate of breast cancer and promoting healthy skin and membranes. I've talked with a number of very athletic women and teens who have cut out the healthy fats because they have been given to understand that all fat is bad. It is no surprise they have stopped menstruating or have other problems with the reproductive system, dry skin, and difficulty in thought processes. Clients who have psoriasis, eczema, and other skin problems have seen excellent results by adding supplemental EFA's along with other nutrients. A good balanced combination is flax / borage. Flax is rich in omega-3 factors, magnesium, potassium and fiber. Black Currant and evening primrose oils contain high amounts of gamma-linoleic acid, with evening primrose containing the highest amount of any food substance. Gamma-linoleic acid is good for the heart, premenstrual syndrome, multiple sclerosis and high blood pressure. It has a positive effect on sex hormone response, including estrogen and testosterone, aids in lowering cholesterol and helps relieve pain and inflammation. Fish oils from salmon, mackerel., herring and sardines are good sources because they have the highest fat content and provide more omega-3 factors than other fishes. Remember, essential fatty acids are called "essential" because we need them. They must be obtained through the foods we eat.

Dyes, Additives, Preservatives

The more a food is processed, the more the nutrients and taste are lost. Manufacturers have "solved?" this problem by adding artificial ingredients. These little chemicals also prolong the shelf life. Dyes, additives and preservatives pose many problems. Artificial sweeteners like aspartame produce side effects in sensitive people. These may be headaches, dizziness, seizures, menstrual problems, mental retardation, behavioral changes and an increased cancer risk, yet it is still popular. We are taking in far more chemicals than you may imagine as reported in Nontoxic, Natural & Earthwise : "The average person in this country consumes five thousand different synthetic chemicals in his or her day-to-day diet for a total of six pounds of preservatives and artificial compounds each year.". . . Of these, it was possible to completely assess the health hazards of only 5 percent. Also, very important is this fact: "Regardless of the results of the toxicity tests for single food additives, the real issue is how they interact, because that is how we consume them. Food additives can have a synergistic effect and become more harmful as they combine." (7)

My son and his friend in Pennsylvania, John Paul, accompanied me to the grocery store for some miscellaneous items one Saturday morning. The boys were thirsty and headed for the beverage aisle. I noticed them in the midst of choosing their drinks. John Paul reached for a "dyed blue" one. I said, "If you can read me the ingredients, it will be my treat." With a grin that lights his entire face, he turned over the bottle and started to read. . The smile soon faded.

"What in the world are all these things, Mrs. Morrone?"

I responded, "The brightly-colored liquids, chartreuse, fluorescent orange and royal blue, of course are not real fruit juices. Those are FD&C dyes in assorted colors and numbers along with artificial sweeteners and other chemicals."

That led to a label reading lesson-- Healthy Foods, Chemicals and Toxins 101 and we settled for a 100% whole apple juice (not from concentrate) and a sparkling water. Upon arriving home, John Paul hurried over to my side of the car. "I'm indebted to you the rest of my life. I will never look at food the same way again!"

Meats and Fish

Meats and fish harbor parasites which are the underlying cause of much illness. Therefore, eating these foods raw or rare increases the risk of transmission. They may also be processed with threatening chemicals such as nitrates and nitrites to prevent spoilage from bacteria. Nitrites cause among a varied list of reactions: lowered blood pressure, headache, dizziness, nausea, visual disturbances, coma and death. Nitrites can also turn into carcinogenic nitrosamines. Meats and fish often contain sodium salts which have been linked to high blood pressure and water retention. Perhaps you've eaten a piece of real salty ham or other luncheon meats and noticed swollen ankles or fingers the next day. Nitrites can deplete our nutritional stores of Vitamin A and interfere with our ability to convert beta-carotene into vitamin A. They can also combine with substances in the proteins we eat call amines.

(7) Non-toxic, Natural & Earthwise, Debra Lynn Dadd.

This combination forms nitrosamines which are cancer-causing. Heterocyclic amines are formed when foods are cooked the wrong way-- high heat, overcooking, charring, grilling and barbecuing. HCA's are molecules that are created when heat breaks up amino acids and creatinine. They promote free radicals, cause DNA mutations, especially in the colon, and target liver, breasts and other organs. Broiling meat does not produce as much of an amine problem as pan frying. HCA's increase with cooking time and increase our cancer risk. Garlic is one food which helps to neutralize these carcinogens. Monosodium glutamate (MSG) is commonly used as a flavor enhancer or tenderizer which has produced many reactions in sensitive individuals from headache, palpitations, weakness to buckling knees and passing out. The FDA lists this additive as one needing further study for its mutagenic effects and possible harm reproductively.

A burger just isn't a burger to many people without processed cheese. Cheese contains preservatives such as BHA/BHT, aerosol propellants, petroleum-based bleaching agents, and residues of hormones, antibiotics and pesticides including DDT. It melts so beautifully because of the aluminum in it. Of course, those burger patties with cheese need to be washed down with a tall, cold soft drink. One of America's favorite soft drinks has an ingredient originally produced as a medicine to suppress the immune system in patients with organ transplants. It has been linked positively to skin cancer. At this point, you are probably thinking nothing that you enjoy is good to eat. You know you need to eat right to be healthy but want to enjoy what you are eating as well. This certainly can be accomplished. How? By consuming foods as close to their natural state as possible, with quality in mind and tastefully prepared. If you eat mostly processed foods, read the labels. Be interested in what you are putting inside your body. If you can't pronounce it, do you want to eat it? I've seen frozen tater tots, and after checking the label, couldn't find any taters in the list of ingredients. On the other hand, there doesn't have to be a long list of unpronounceable ingredients on a carrot, celery, pear, cucumber or apple, and if it says "organic", that is a great benefit. These foods are what they are while grown in healthier conditions. When foods are conventionally grown, we should demand to know whether or not they have been genetically-modified or irradiated. We already know they have pesticide residues.

Refined White Flour/Sugar

This section will be short and sweet, no pun intended. Refined white flour and refined sugar are dead foods. Flour starts out with about 30 different nutrients, and by the time its done its refining process, there are virtually none left. Seven or eight are added back and it is called "enriched". Sugar, unbelievably, is in so many processed foods. You'll find it in a can of peas, corn, ketchup, tortilla chips, bread, crackers, soup, dressings and spaghetti sauce. Read labels, you'll be surprised. White flour and sugar require large amounts of pancreatic enzymes to digest them. The pancreas works overtime, can become disabled and under-produces necessary enzymes for digestion. Enzyme insufficiency can cause degenerative conditions. Refined sugar contributes to hypoglycemia, candida, adrenal exhaustion, high cholesterol, immune disorders, and many other imbalances. Healthy alternatives to these two impoverished foods are 100% whole grain flours such as oat, barley, wheat, kamut, rice, rye, spelt, corn, and buckwheat. Complex sweeteners such as date sugar, barley malt, and brown rice syrup are much preferred for their nutritional content.

For those who cannot tolerate sugar due to blood sugar imbalances, the herb stevia or honeyleaf from South America is a great treasure. It is a naturally sweet, nutritious herb that is helpful in nourishing the pancreas and doesn't affect blood sugar levels. This comes in liquid, powder and chopped leaves. It is non-caloric and excellent for weight loss.

Preparation

Thoroughly wash fruits and vegetables. Most people know they need to adequately cook their meats, but I've seen folks tear the cellophane off a head of lettuce, break it up in a salad bowl, and pour dressing on it. I've also seen it rinsed off under tap water and eaten. Remember, produce grown in fertilizers and handled by humans, can be contaminated with bacteria. Tap water itself may contain bacteria. If the food can be washed, wash it. There are effective fruit and veggie washes available at health food stores and larger, more health conscious food chains. It's well worth the investment to avoid bouts with parasites and other infections.

Eating all cooked foods poses additional problems. Cooking can destroy most of the health-promoting enzymes. Our bodies have over 2700 different types of enzymes performing complicated tasks at lightening speeds. Enzymes are necessary for each biochemical reaction in the body, and we only have so many at birth. We do not continue to replenish them as we live and age. When foods are eaten that contain their own enzymes intact, they aid our digestive processes. Cooking also destroys vitamins B and C. Estimates have been given on nutrient losses from foods. The chart below gives an idea of how much nutrients are lost. (This comes from a clipping in my files, and I apologize that I cannot remember its source.)

Cooked fresh	56% are lost in cooking
Canned	30% are lost in the scalding process
	25% in the liquid diffusion
	12% in reheating
Frozen	25% in the scalding process
	19% in freezing
	5% in thawing
	24% in cooking

Eating a higher percentage of foods in their raw state as they would come from the garden, will give us the maximum amount of nutrition from whole food sources. Buy your produce as fresh as possible, and be mindful how it is stored. Carefully examine for bruises, brown spots, mushiness or soft, moldy spots. These are indicative that the produce is old or has been sitting too long unrefrigerated

It is important to eat a variety of foods. Americans commonly consume 25% dairy, 25% meat and poultry, 25% wheat products and the remaining percentages from sugar, fat and small amounts of fruits and vegetables. The "I'll have a burger, fries and soft drink" pretty much says it all. To merely eat from the basic food groups is not the answer. It's the quality, quantity and variety that we must consider.

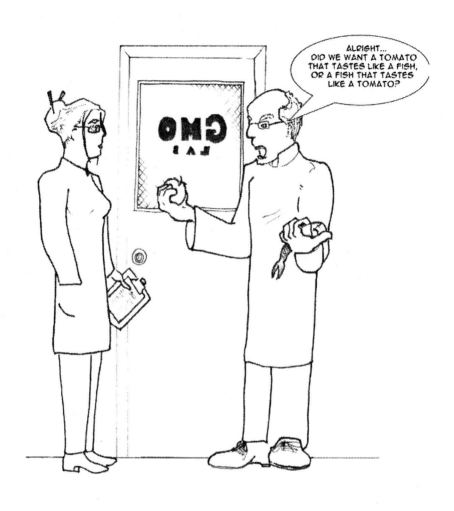

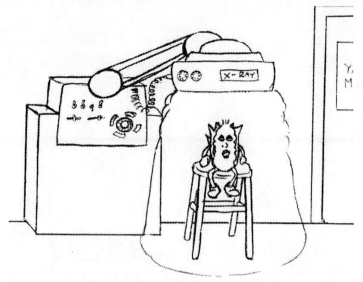

"OKAY MR. KORN.
TAKE A DEEP BREATH...HOLD IT!"

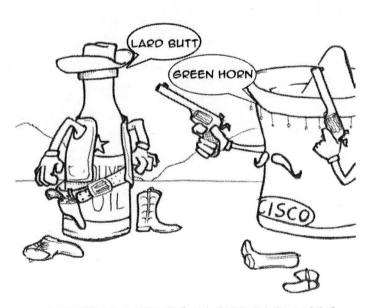

FIGHTING WORDS IN THE FATLANDS

Part Two:
Just For the Health of It

CHAPTER FIVE

QUALITY FOODS FOR LIFE

I've finally found why babies suck their thumbs. I tried some of the baby food.

The World's All-time Best Collection of Good Clean Jokes by Bob Phillips

Life in the Soil

Have you ever stood at the edge of a large field of corn? It's impossible to discern the incalculable number of plants growing there, sometimes as far as the eye can see. Regardless of the stage of growth, one invariably begins to picture the harvest. Those big, golden ears of corn on the cob will be prepared to perfection, and savored with mouthwatering delight. We usually don't appreciate all the behind the scene activity in those fields in order for the fruits of the earth to be enjoyed.

The ecosystems-- communities of plants, animals and microorganisms-- are interacting with one another and their environments, and they are interdependent on each other for survival. As an example, Dr. Sara Wright of the US Department of Agriculture, identified the role played by mycorrhizal fungi in the soil:

"She discovered that these fungi produce glomalin, a protein that contributes to soil fertility by facilitating the aggregation of fine soil particles. Glomalin, as it was named by Dr. Wright, has also been called soil superglue. Pesticides can interfere with glomalin production. Mycorrhizal fungi living within the root cells of plants can be harmed by fungicides or indirectly by herbicides which poison the host plant." (8)

Knowing the role our food plays in healing and longevity, we should understand why a healthful growing process in that ecosystem is so important.

Organic Farming

Plants do more than merely standing in dirt and sunbathing waiting to be picked. They also eat and drink. With the help of soil-based organisms, they take up inorganic nutrients through their root systems, and change them into the organic nutrients we require for life. Green plants also convert the energy in sunlight into chemical energy by locking it within the bonds of synthesized food molecules. So, what plants eat, good or poor, feeds us. It stands to reason that plants raised without "time bomb" ingredients such as chemical fertilizers, pesticides, and nuclear radiation are going to be much more nutritious and vital to us.

Natural farming methods produce healthy, organically-grown foods. Organic farming as practiced from inception uses no synthetic chemicals and works with the natural environment, not against it. The soil must be conditioned with additives such as mineral rich seaweed fertilizers, rock dust or stone meal, colloidal soft rock phosphate and composted organic matter. Organic growing invites beneficial insects such as ladybugs and green lacewings to the garden to keep harmful species in check, and does companion planting and crop rotation to disrupt disease and pest life cycles. It uses animal manures, compost and cover crops instead of fertilizer squeezed from Persian Gulf crude petroleum or human waste. There are no "estrogenic pesticides" (xenoestrogens) that influence abnormal sexual development in animals and humans or mimic human estrogen to drive cancers. It puts nutrients back into the soil that the next crop will feed upon and in turn give to us nourishing food.

---

(8) Rachel Carson Council News No. 91, Spring 1999, page 5, 5-d "Effects on Beneficial Mycorrhizal Fungi...."

Threats and Compromises

Within the past ten years, the words "natural" and "organic" were continually at risk for being watered down and seriously compromised. Attempts surfaced from large Agribusiness through legislative bills and lobbyists to change the traditional meaning of organic to include sewage sludge as fertilizer and a host of other "compromises". After much debate and painstaking deliberation, the Secretary of Agriculture introduced on December 20, 2000, a 500-page document of "the strongest and most comprehensive organic standard in the world." Efforts are still ongoing, however, to weaken this.

Beyond the beauty of organic farming is Biodynamic organic farming that recognizes the basic principles at work in nature to bring about balance and healing. Biodyamics, founded in 1924 by Austrian-born scientist and philosopher, Dr. Rudolf Steiner, is a holistic system of farming and gardening which regards the earth as a living organism. It considers the interrelationship of all the kingdoms, mineral, plant, animal and human, in the ecosystem and how they correspond to the rhythms and activities of the greater universe. It strives to renew the soil with life-sustaining properties to produce food full of vitality, rich in nutritients. It requires the careful observance of nature to determine the best growing conditions for the best yield-- shade or full sun, wet or dry, how solar, lunar and planetary rhythms affect growth and growing times. For more information on biodynamic farms, write to Bio-Dynamic Farming and Gardening Association, Inc., P. O. Box 550, Kimberton, PA 19442 or Applied Bio-Dynamics, Inc., P. O. Box 133, Woolwine, VA 24185-0133.

Though it may not be possible to have your our own biodynamic farm or organic garden, it is advantageous to buy certified organic as much as possible to lessen the amount of toxic chemical exposure through foods as well as optimizing nutritional benefit. Look for "Certified Organic" or "Demeter Certified Organic" labels. (Demeter Association represents Bio-dynamic agriculture.) This is quality food for the health of it, to sustain our lives and flourish.

Meat

On the high cost of meat, PREVENTIVE MEDICINE, November 1995, reported: "U. S. health care costs could be reduced by $29 billion to $61 billion a year if Americans cut meat out of their diet, according to researchers from the Physicians' Committee for Responsible Medicine."

The committee is a Washington-based organization promoting vegetarianism. They further added: "The health effects of an omnivorous diet may result in the presence of meat, the displacement of plant foods or both." In every study of large groups of US populations they examined, meat eaters were more likely to suffer serious health problems. In an accompanying editorial, two of the doctors wrote: "The combined medical costs attributable to smoking and meat consumption exceed the predicted costs of providing health coverage for all currently uninsured Americans."

Meat will add higher fat, saturated fat, and higher calories to a diet. If you choose to eat meat, fish and poultry, certified organic is a guarantee that the products are hormone free, additive, preservative, pesticide and antibiotic free. The animal has been fed organic feed. Free range means the animal was not raised in overcrowded, unsanitary and sickly conditions, but allowed to roam and graze.

Fruits and Vegetables

Many individuals have opted for a vegetarian diet for health as well as other reasons. There are numerous books and cookbooks on the subject of vegetarianism. Just a little side story-- I had to attend a parent-teacher conference. After finding out about my work, my daughter's teacher proudly told me her daughter is a vegetarian. I asked her to elaborate on what she eats each day. Apparently, she opens a can of peas, corn and beans for an after school meal. She will have a can of vegetable soup for dinner, and for breakfast some toast and coffee. Perhaps there is an occasional salad at school. That's pretty much it-- every day. Although the concept was there, the practice obviously was not healthy. We already considered nutrient loss in the canning process and reheating. If the can is not lead free and specially coated, the leaching of lead, aluminum and other metals takes place into the food.

Obviously quality whole, living foods combined properly to get complete proteins are the healthy vegetarian approach. You may, however, need to supplement B 12 since it is found largely in animal food sources. Combining foods properly entails learning what foods complement each other. It's a good idea to eat fruits separately; they're enzyme-rich requiring less digestive time in the stomach before they begin to break down and move on. They also can speed up metabolism due to their high sugar content. Fresh fruits are high in natural water, are cleansing to the system, alkalizing, and contain many vitamins and other nutrients. They serve us best when eaten alone. Once cooked, they become acid-forming in the body. It's a good idea to eat melons by themselves as they digest very rapidly. When eaten at the end of a meal or with other foods, fruits start to ferment since they are held back in the digestive process. One may experience gas, bloating or other discomfort. In general, proteins combine well with vegetables. Vegetables combine well with grains and starches.

Juicing For Vibrant Health

In Chapter Two, we discussed how the primary cause of every sickness and disease is toxemia and malnutrition. Addressing nutritional deficiencies with such elements as vitamins, organic minerals and salts will help achieve a better quality of health. Fresh raw vegetables, fruits, seeds, sprouts and nuts, are live, health-building foods because every atom in their composition is infused with life-promoting enzymes.

Fresh organic fruit and vegetable juice is one of the most effective, valuable ways take advantage of their benefits. Juicing should separate the distilled water, vital elements and precious enzymes in the food from the fiber. We may juice eight to ten whole carrots but we certainly wouldn't eat that much fiber at one sitting. There is virtually no nourishment in the fiber. The juice, will be speedily digested in just a matter of ten to fifteen minutes, without taxing the digestive organs or using up energy in the process. The enzymes and other nutrients are absorbed readily, nourishing the cells and tissues of the body. This is why you will feel an immediate energy boost when you need it. When one is ill or if there are chewing or digestive problems, the therapeutic benefits of vegetables and fruits are easily obtained this way. Eating them in whole form requires hours of digestive activity before the nutrients finally reach the cells and tissues. We still need to eat plenty of raw foods each day for the fiber as well as for all their other properties. Fiber serves as an intestinal broom. Since pesticides and toxins are stored in the fiber, it is definitely healthier to eat organically grown.

Blenders, liquefiers, and food processors are unable to extract juice from fruits and vegetables. Therapeutic juicing requires an appliance that separates the juice from the pulp. Numerous inefficient "entry-level" juicers flood the market. There are effective fruit and vegetable juicers, wheat grass juicers and combination juicers. Hydraulic press / triturator types are most effective, though quite expensive. For home use, a centrifugal juice extractor with functional parts comprised of surgical steel will last for many years. By lining the vertical basket with paper filters, no fibers seep into the juice and cleanup is relatively easy.

Let's look more closely at the benefits of fresh fruits and vegetables. The National Cancer Institute has published much data relative to the potential of phytochemicals (Phyto meaning plant-based.) There are literally tens of thousands of these in the foods we eat, and mostly all are found in our fruits and veggies. Here are just some that have been identified:

❖ D-glucarate found in apples, oranges, grapefruits, brussels sprouts and broccoli, helps support and protect our body's ability to detox carcinogens by combining them with water-soluble substances.

❖ Alpha Carotene and Beta Carotene are carotenoids found in cantaloupe, carrots, red and yellow peppers, pumpkin, apricots, sweet potatoes, spinach and other leafy greens. They are converted into Vitamin A in the liver. They are antioxidants, helping to protect the cells against cancer and other diseases.

❖ Bioflavonoids are not produced within the human body, but must be obtained through foods such as onions, buckwheat, and most fruits. Besides enhancing the absorption of Vitamin C, they work synergistically with C to strengthen capillaries, blood vessels and promote circulation. They reduce pain, bumps and bruises, have an antibacterial effect, help lower cholesterol, stimulate bile production, and help prevent cataracts.

❖ Cryptoxanthin - food carotene found in peaches, tangerines, oranges, papaya, and nectarines.

❖ Lutein - is a nutrient from carotenoids but not converted to Vitamin A. It does serve as a potent antioxidant.

❖ Lutein and Zeaxanthin, lends the most support to the eyes as they make up the yellow pigment in the retina and appear to specifically

provide protection to the macula. These are
and other fruits and vegetables.

❖ Indole 3-Carbinol - found in cabbage, col.
cruciferous vegetables which possess protective
health-promoting benefits at cellular level. It reduce.
of mammary cancers. Cabbage juice also contains
which is very healing to ulcers.

❖ Lycopene is a red carotenoid found in tomatoes, watermelon, guava
and apricots. It may protect against cancer growth and induce
apoptosis-- the natural programmed death of cells.

❖ Ellagic Acid is a cancer-preventing compound found in
strawberries, red raspberries and other fruits. It binds to carcinogens
and renders them inactive. It has also been shown to provide
protection against chromosomal damage and breaks in the DNA
strands in lymphocytes exposed to radiation.

❖ Sulforaphane found in broccoli and other cruciferous vegetables,
helps mobilize the body's natural fighting resources and reduces the
risk of developing cancer. It can block the formation of tumors
from chemical carcinogens and has demonstrated to induce
apoptosis.

❖ Isoflavones such as genistein and daidzein found in soybeans are
flavonoids that inhibit DNA oxidative damage. They protect cells
against irregular growth from multiple unique organisms as in
carcinogenesis.

❖ Apigenin is found in celery, basil, artichokes, parsley, alfalfa and
other plants. It is the most effective anti-proliferative flavonoid
tested. It prevents over proliferation of cancer cells in response to
estrogen by binding to estrogen receptor sites on the cell membrane.
(Many cancers are estrogen-driven.)

❖ Reservatrol has been shown to inhibit platelet aggregation-- a
clumping together of blood cells which can result from spending
alot of time in front of your computer. This anti-oxidant is found in
the skin of grapes and red wine.

❖ Polyacetylenes found in parsley, carrots and celery, protect against
certain carcinogens found in tobacco smoke and help regulate
prostaglandins.

..oids prevent dental decay and act as an anti-ulcer agent.
, bind to estrogen and inhibit cancer by suppressing unwanted
enzyme activity. Citrus fruits, licorice root and soy products contain
triterpenoids.

❖ Canima-glutamylallylic cysteines are found in aged garlic extract
and may have a role in lowering blood pressure and elevating
immune system activities.

How Can We Not Like Them?

When you think about it, man is delving into, inspecting and
discovering these and other unique properties within something from
nature, be it herb or food. The isolation of a single nutrient and
discovery of its implications to health are both exciting and mind-
staggering. It is seen as nothing less than a miracle, but the race is then
on to produce and duplicate this isolated find into a breakthrough
designer drug. How many other undiscovered miracles are
synergistically contained in perfect balance in that self-same living
food? Appreciating this beautiful synergy, there are many individuals
who will only eat raw, living foods because of the obvious health
benefits. Fresh fruits and raw vegetables give us the nutrients and
properties we need that are life-sustaining. They facilitate
detoxification and removal of substances which are dangerous to the
body. The phytochemicals they contain will obviously help block the
effect of undesirable, toxic chemicals from becoming cancer-
promoters. We in natural health appreciate that cancer cells need an
environment in which to attach, grow and proliferate. Our lifestyles
largely determine whether this environment is a favorable or
unfavorable one.

Incorporate a salad every day if you have not been a vegetable fan
up to now and try to select a nice variety of them. Remember, when
you want to cook your vegetables in addition to eating them raw, light
steaming will preserve as many nutrients as possible. By changing over
to a healthier diet, our taste buds will more acutely appreciate the
wholesome taste of foods that are healing and nutrient-dense. When the
cravings for sugar, salt, fats and artificial flavors are present, healthy
foods usually do not have as much appeal. Also, smoking, over-
consumption of alcohol and the aforementioned things, reduce our
nutrient stores and result in impaired senses of taste and smell.

When Foods Do Not Agree

Processed foods, over-chemicalized and enzyme depleted, cause our bodies to assume full digestive responsibilities. Digestion eventually weakens over time, which results in larger-sized particles of undigested fats and proteins entering the bloodstream. They are now perceived as foreign bodies or toxins to our immune system, and an allergic reaction may occur. As the total burden of toxins increase, we become less tolerant to even minute amounts of any allergen.

Besides eating chemically-altered or processed foods which we are not able to handle, other common causes of food sensitivities or intolerances stem from a system too alkaline with low gastric pH, lack of sleep, chronic infections, emotional upsets, and enzyme deficiencies. When our bodies detox sufficiently and other imbalances are corrected, digestion and assimilation usually improve. Imbalances may negate the use of certain foods. For example, an underactive thyroid would not do well on "goitrogens"-- foods that prevent the use of iodine. These are cabbage, peanuts, millet, turnips, soy products, broccoli, mustard greens, spinach, and kale. If eaten raw, eat them in moderation. Cooking inactivated the goitrogens. Also, one with candida albicans or yeast problems, does well to stay away from foods which feed the yeasts such as all simple carbohydrates-- white flour products and sugars, as well as fermented foods and foods containing yeast.

There are many other conditions which could be considered here, but as we discussed earlier, each one is biochemically unique. Diets really should be individualized based upon one's needs and health goals. A professional schooled and experienced in holistic nutrition will be extremely valuable to you.

So, What Do I Eat?

Savor the flavor and feel immense satisfaction from the succulent goodness of whole, organically-grown foods. Try to select the freshest possible and take advantage of the fruits and vegetables in season that are locally grown. Don't be bashful about asking the produce manager in your supermarket to special order for you, or try to locate a "co-op" in your area.

Prepare your foods artistically and creatively with fresh herbs and spices for meal presentations truly worth remembering. A little extra effort will bring compliments at the dinner table. These are the quality foods-- for life! The question now is, will our excellent diet give us all we need?

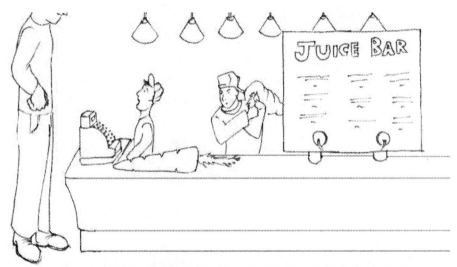

"SO THATS ONE EXTRA-LARGE CARROT JUICE?"

CHAPTER SIX

SUPPLEMENTING YOUR FOOD

A customer called one of the
health food stores
where I worked some years ago.
She said she was all out of her Vitamin B 12's.
She wanted to know if she could take two B 6's.

Susanne

It Was The Best of Times, It's now the Toxic Times

After reading Chapter Four, it's pretty obvious our food chain is in big trouble. In order to maintain health and well-being, the human body requires a number of nutrients in greater or lesser amounts depending upon individual needs. Exercising heavily and frequently increases our nutrient requirements. Illness along with taking regular medications may call for a number of nutrients in therapeutic amounts to replenish our stores and rebuild health. Years of bad habits such as using tobacco, alcohol, drugs and a poor diet have likely caused deficits in precious nutrients. Abundant chemicals in the environment adversely affect our nutritional stores depending upon the type and amount of exposure and how well our detoxification processes are working. The average person is not aware of the daily toxic exposure.

I recently found out about a pesticide soil drench procedure in new home construction. Approximately 200 gallons of pesticide saturates the soil just prior to pouring the concrete foundation. Residents of that new home would have to contend with vapors finding their way into indoor air for literally years and years after application.

Nursery schools, preschools and public schools are usually built on land situated in close proximity to high-tension wires and substations. Subsequently, our children are exposed to high-risk EMF's (electromagnetic frequencies) which have been shown to cause leukemia, tumors and many forms of cancer. Studies also have been conducted with electromagnetic fields from VDT's (video display terminals) contributing to visual system dysfunction, musculoskeletal disorders, stress and adverse pregnancy outcomes such as reduced birth weight, pre-term birth and spontaneous abortion. Radon is common in many parts of the country, seeping up through the ground and into our homes. Highly-toxic molds and mildews are becoming more prevalent in the news. Once a serious toll is imposed on the immune system, greater nutritional support is vital. How would we even suspect an environmental culprit to be the cause of our health problems unless we become aware that these dangers exist? It takes concern, asking questions and educating ourselves. Contrary to that old saying, ignorance is not bliss.

Soil Quality A Factor

Although fruits and vegetables are vital to health, few eat a sufficient amount of them on a daily basis. Another problem is the quality of the soil in which our food is grown. The soil is supposed to contain minerals, plants uptake those minerals, and we eat the plants. In other words, the inorganic minerals in the soil are transformed into an organic form which we can absorb and assimilate. Way back in 1936, the US government published a paper exposing the fact that our soils were severely depleted of minerals. How did this happen?

Farmers in past centuries made it a practice to allow dead fields to rest so that wildlife and rotting plants could restore the land's fertility. Modern technology came along and completely ignored this important ecological necessity. Over sixty years have passed from the publishing of that government paper, and the situation has only gotten worse by dumping environmentally-destructive pesticides and chemicals into the soil. These kill the soil-based organisms vital to the soil quality and utilization of minerals by plants. So, rather than waiting for our bodies to break down from nutritional deficiencies, we must supplement our diet with the proper superfoods, vitamins, minerals, etc.

Is The RDA Enough?

Nutritional experts all agree that there is basic nutrition to stave off such diseases as scurvy, beri beri, rickets, and night blindness. The RDA (recommended dietary allowances) was created over forty years ago, using these minimums as a standard preventative daily intake. In today's world, we need optimal or beyond basic nutrition, not minimums. The cleaner we live, the more effective our bodies are at cleansing, the better the diet, then the less supplementation we may need. This must be true since peoples in other parts of the world living with healthier conditions (mineral-rich soil, cleaner air, fresh-grown foods and less stress) have longevity well beyond the average American. Any regimen of optimal supplementation should be individualized or customized by a nutritionally-oriented health professional.

But My Doctor Says. . .

Your doctor may have already told you supplements are a bunch of bunk! This comment is usually followed by "Just eat a balanced diet from the basic food groups." We've already looked at our food situation. The medical community's focus has been and for the most part, still is on medicine. Therefore, the bias fuels the comments. They acquire proficiency and excellence in their respective fields of medicine, including the study of drugs. Supplements are not drugs. They do not have the side effects of drugs nor the potential to kill you by serious interactions. Many negative reports in the media regarding nutritional supplements are from questionable products which I would call the "fringe" of the industry. These may contain unhealthy stimulants, poor quality although natural ingredients, herbs not in keeping with traditional herbal medicine use, artificial ingredients and additives, and even recreational drugs under the guise of dietary supplements. When considering weight loss products containing stimulants such as ephedrine, caffeine and perhaps designer street drugs: Caveat Emptor-- Let the Buyer Beware.

There are occasions when taking both supplements and drugs calls for caution. For example, your doctor may have you taking Heparin (an anticoagulant drug). Vitamin E and C are effective at helping to thin the blood, so these along with the drug would not be advisable. Individuals who have organ transplants and are on immune-suppressant drugs, are told not to take supplements which boost immune activity. I have always found juicing and superfoods to be very beneficial in these cases. It bears repeating; we need expert guidance to use supplements therapeutically or when taking prescription drugs.

On occasion, individuals who have allergies to dust, molds and pollens may have a negative reaction to herbs. A good rule of thumb is to begin any new herb at one-fourth the recommended dosage. Working closely with your health care provider, choosing the right herb will be less likely a problem. Taking herbs while pregnant should not be done unless under the direction of your doctor or other qualified health care professional. Many herbs are contraindicated in pregnancy. Herbal beverage teas are usually fine. You may have a negative attitude about supplements in general because of a lack of experience with them, or you may have taken them for a time and not noticed any appreciable difference. There are many things to consider when taking supplements. It is important to get good quality ingredients, the right form for maximum absorption, and know the amount that is necessary for your needs. There are capsules, tablets, lozenges, liquids, powders, sublinguals, sprays and inter-nasals. Some supplements have a "shellac" coating that is very difficult to break down. They are often seen passing through into the toilet bowl just as they went in. Minerals are difficult to digest and absorb depending upon their form. Synthetic minerals, such as iron (ferrous sulfate) may cause constipation and nausea. Some inorganic calcium supplements such as dolomite or oyster shell are fossilized rocks. These can be utilized well by your plants but may not be digested, absorbed and assimilated well in humans. Malabsorption is a common problem, so choosing the most absorbable form of the supplement along with some digestive enzymes would be logical.

There's an explosion of interest in supplements akin to the "Gold rush". Many new companies are springing up in hopes of grabbing a share of a huge and skyrocketing industry. Advertisers without a natural foods or scientific background bombard the marketplace. You wonder if quality and integrity are intact. Ingredients may not match the label, so read labels carefully. "Natural" doesn't necessarily mean all the ingredients are natural. It may say all natural ginseng, which can simply mean the ginseng is natural but the other ingredients aren't. There may be artificial colors, preservatives, coal tars, mica, talc, sugars, starch and other additives. We certainly don't need to supplement our food with more synthetic chemicals. Scrutinize the labels the same way you do food and beverages.

It is wise to do some research on the products you'll be incorporating in your program to be sure to get maximum nutritional benefit. A balanced program may consist of individual vitamins, minerals, herbs, and/or amino acids, as well as nutrient-rich, superfood supplements. Superfoods include cereal grasses, bee products, sea vegetation, soy lecithin, fish oils, etc. They provide complete nutrition in their natural state, easy to digest and assimilate, rich in antioxidants, enzymes, essential fatty acids, vitamins, a variety of minerals, and high-quality proteins. The nice thing to appreciate about superfoods is that they are made by God in nature, and not by man in laboratories.

More on Safety

What about safety? Those not familiar with therapeutic benefits of nutritional supplements may be thrust in opposing directions like the pendulum of a clock. One minute the media reports it's a miracle supplement, and the next minute its a dangerous substance ready to be pulled from the shelves. This is usually the case when the latest study is reported in the news. Vitamins A, C, Beta Carotene, tryptophan, chaparral, phenylalanine, ephedra all have been in the spotlight. It is important to find out exactly how the study was done, what the parameters were, how the conclusions were drawn, and what other studies may refute these findings. If an individual is harmed, what are the circumstances?

Several years ago a study was published that long-term smokers had a slightly greater risk of developing lung cancer if taking beta carotene supplements. It's quite interesting that the same study concluded that these smokers had better lung function with beta carotene and those who previously smoked had a lower risk of lung cancer on beta carotene. Further analysis revealed that beta carotene reduced the risk of prostate cancer among this group of smokers provided they didn't drink alcohol. Usually, when an item is reported in the news, it doesn't always cover the whole story and may in fact present a biased view.

ECHINACEA

Mark Blumenthal, in WHOLE FOODS MAGAZINE of January, 1999, wrote an article entitled "Echinacea Study Misreported in Press". He explained how the mass media misreported the results of a clinical study on the herb, echinacea. The study was reported to show a lack of cold-preventive effects while the authors of the study reinforced cold treatment benefits. The article clearly outlined the efficacy and use of echinacea as well as documented studies and research results. I like the conclusion drawn by publisher Jack Challem of the NUTRITION REPORTER, on this back and forth, seesaw reporting: "Bad studies may be more dangerous than vitamins."

In the March, 2002, issue of NATURAL FOOD MERCHANDISER, page 32, an article entitled "Echinacea May Cause Allergic Reactions" by Wendy L. Bonifazi, R.N., reported on a study published in the 2002 issue of Annals of Allergy, Asthma and Immunology. This study was conducted in Austrailia and "based upon observed reactions in five patients referred to the researchers for evaluation, and 51 adverse reaction reports submitted to the Austrailian Adverse Drug Reactions Advisory Committee. They involved at least six different brands of echinacea in the form of tea, tablets and liquid. The five observed cases reacted with acute asthma attacks, shock, skin rash, burning throat, chest pains hives, diarrhea, facial and airway swelling, dizziness and disorientation." The article pointed out "Echinacea is a member of the Asteraceae family including such plants as ragweed, mugwort, sagebrush, chrysanthemums, marigolds" and various other flowers.

Allergic reactions to this degree have not been reported in the United States. Individuals can have hypersensitive reactions to various plants. Herbs, however, are used by millions of people worldwide, and the study presents a few cases. Even with the upsurge in large numbers of those taking herbs for the first time, the problems that occur annually are quite low. This is hardly the case with reactions to over-the-counter or prescribed conventional drugs. Echinacea is not typically used for allergies anyway, but rather for its effecting a variety of viral and bacterial conditions. It boosts the immune system, increasing production of white blood cells. It is considered one of the best blood cleansers and purifiers. Since allergies are triggered by a hypersensitive immune response, it wouldn't be logical to use an immune system stimulant such as echinacea for allergies or asthma.

VITAMIN C

I heard years ago from my family practitioner that "vitamin C causes kidney stones". This bit of information surfaces from time to time, especially if it's brought up during the medical exam. Skeptics claim that large amounts of C could promote stones due to the fact that when ascorbic acid is broken down, one of its byproducts is oxalate. Oxalates combine with calcium in the urine to form calcium-oxalate kidney stones. The amount of oxalates produced by vitamin C is very small even when taking megadoses.

Doctors and other health professionals who routinely tell their patients to take vitamin C for long periods of time do not report that stones are common. Further studies indicate that vitamin C can help lower the risk of stones. (9)

L-Tryptophan

When the subject of tryptophan comes up, many people don't understand why it was banned since it was a staple in their supplement regimen for years to promote calmness and sleep. People died from taking tryptophan as reported in the news. What happened to cause the FDA's banning of L-Tryptophan, is, I believe, one story worth your full attention. When the facts start unfolding, it is material prime for a Hollywood movie not any less spectacular than Silkwood, Erin Brockovitch, China Syndrome or All the President's Men. The Center

---

(9) Journal of Urology 1996, 155: 1847-1851; January, 1996 issue of Nutrition and Healing)

for Disease Control in 1989 reported evidence linking L-Tryptophan supplements to eosinophilia myalgia, a blood disorder characterized by elevated white blood cells. There was at least one death resulting from this illness. Although the cause of EMS is still unknown, the FDA recalled all products in which L-Tryptophan is a major ingredient and banned its sale in the US on March 22, 1990. This ban continues today.

The best recap I have come across is a concise report written by Dr. Dean Wolfe Manders, a senior lecturer in humanities and sciences at the California College of Arts and Crafts, Oakland/San Francisco. Dr. Manders did extensive research on the medical politics of L-Tryptophan. His enlightening report entitled "The FDA Ban of L.-Tryptophan: Politics, Profits and Prozac Social Policy, Vol. 26, No. 2, Winter 1995" appears on the worldwide web on a number of web sites. Please check these out and read the comments in their entirety:

http://www.lef.org/fda/fdaban95.html;
http://www.lightparty.com/indexhtml>;
http://www.copi.com/articles_tryptophan.

For those of you who may not have access to the Web, I'll highlight some of his salient points:

~March 26, 1990, NEWSWEEK featured a lead article praising the virtues of "Prozac: A Breakthrough Drug for Depression". The FDA ban of L-Tryptophan and the Newsweek Prozac story occurred within four days of each other, unnoticed by both the media and public. Yet to those who understand the effective properties of L-Tryptophan and Prozac, the concurrence seems unbelievably coincidental. Prozac and other new antidepressant drugs attempt to enhance levels of serotonin whereas L-Tryptophan is much more effective as a serotonin producer. The millions of Americans who for decades safely had relied upon L-Tryptophan to relieve depression, anxiety and PMS, control pain and induce natural sleep, have been forced elsewhere for solutions. Routinely such solutions are pharmaceutical in nature: people are driven either to use drugs that are often highly addictive, expensive and sometimes dangerous,......... or simply to suffer.

~Present FDA public policy maintains that it is an untested, unapproved and hazardous drug. The Mayo Clinic and CDC did analytical research a few years ago which traced the fall 1989 outbreak of the serious flu-like condition to contaminants found in batches of L-Tryptohan made by the Japanese Pharmaceutical company, Showa Denko. Yet, this has not convinced the FDA to allow it back on the market. The FDA and NIMH scientists state that irrespective of contaminants, its still a dangerous substance. Other university-based research scientists disagree with these findings.

❖ On February 9, 1993, a US government patent (#518517) was issued to use L-Tryptophan to treat and cure EMS, the very same deadly flu-like condition that prompted the FDA to take L-Tryptophan off the market in 1989.

❖ Notwithstanding its public ban and import alert on L-Tryptophan, the FDA allows Ajinomoto USA the right to import from Japan human-use L-Tryptophan. It is distributed through the Ajinomoto plant in Raleigh, NC, then sold to a network of compounding pharmacies across the US. It is now a high-priced prescription drug in the serotonin marketplace, about 100 capsules for approximately $75 (far more than the cost of the dietary supplement).

❖ During and after the 1989 outbreak, the FDA did not totally ban the use of L-Tryptophan in humans- then, as today, the FDA has granted the pharmaceutical industry the protected right to use L-Tryptophan in hospital settings.

❖ The USDA still sanctions the legal sale and use of non-contaminated L-Tryptophan for animals. There is feed grade L-Tryptophan used as a nutritional and bulk-feed additive, and it is available for use by veterinarians in caring for horses and pets. It's never been removed from baby food produced and sold within the US.

❖ L-Tryptophan is widely used outside the US in Canada, the Netherlands, Germany and England. Nowhere have any serious or widespread health problems been reported.

❖ At bottom, the FDA public ban of safe, non-contaminated L-Tryptophan is uneven, expensive and biased in favor of the pharmaceutical industry. The FDA proscription effectively awards billions of dollars in profits to pharmaceutical companies and their suppliers in the same proportion as it adds billions of unnecessary dollars to the nation's already bloated health care expenditures.

❖ The FDA has succeeded in carrying out its stated policy goal. With competition from publicly available L-Tryptophan removed, the rapidly expanding market in prescription serotonin drugs- now among them L-Tryptophan itself - contains no major "discentives" for the massive accumulation of pharmaceutical industry profits.... The story of L-Tryptophan illustrates a sad and perverse picture of the politics and priorities of public health in America. A safe, dietary-supplement serotonin producer is publicly unavailable to people, while daily fed to animals by corporate agribusiness. A drug patent is approved to use L-Tryptophan to cure the very condition the FDA claims it caused. And, while publicly exclaiming that L-Tryptophan is a dangerous and untested drug, the FDA quietly allows human-use L-Tryptophan to be imported and then marketed and sold by the pharmaceutical industry. To allow the FDA ban on L-Tryptophan to continue unreviewed and uninvestigated condemns millions of Americans to unnecessary financial expenditures and needless suffering.

Along with this information, from the National Eosinophilia Myalgia Syndrome Network website, www.nemsn.org/medical.htm, comes further revealing eye openers from John B. Fagan, PhD., Professor of Molecular Biology of Maharishi University of Management, Iowa, in his article "Summary of the Tryptophan Toxicity Incident". Again, some highlights of his report:

❖ Amino acids are often manufactured by fermentative processes, in which large quantities of bacteria are grown in vats, and the food supplement is extracted from the bacteria and purified. Tryptophan has been produced in this way for many years. In the late 1980's Showa Denko K.K. decided to use genetic engineering to accelerate and increase the efficiency of the production process. They genetically engineered bacteria by inserting new genes that caused the bacteria to express new enzymes. The enzymes were not present in massive amounts, but they altered the cellular metabolism substantially, leading to greatly increased production of tryptophan.

❖ These genetically engineered bacteria were immediately used in commercial production of tryptophan, and the product placed on the market in the USA in 1988. The FDA allowed Showa Denko to sell this genetically engineered product without testing. It was argued that the method of production (whether natural or genetically engineered bacteria) was immaterial and that, since tryptophan had already been shown to be safe, the new material needed no testing. FDA regulations did not require that the new tryptophan be labeled as genetically engineered. This product was placed on the market, and within three months, 37 people died and 1500 were permanently disabled from using this product. It took months to discover that the poisoning was due to the presence of traces of a toxic contaminant in the new genetically engineered tryptophan. One factor that contributed to the time delay was the fact that the product was not labeled as genetically engineered.

❖ It was later shown that the genetically engineered tryptophan contained a highly toxic contaminant comprising less than 0.1% of the total weight of the product, yet it was enough to kill people. . . .It appears that genetic manipulations led to increased tryptophan biosynthesis, which led to increased cellular levels of tryptophan and precursors. At these high levels, these compounds reacted with themselves, generating a deadly toxin.

❖ Some ambiguity remains regarding this incident because it was quite threatening to a number of parties, including Showa Denko, the FDA, the biotechnology industry, and the food supplement industry.. . Showa Denko was vulnerable to legal action (and eventually paid more than one billion dollars to victims and their survivors). The FDA was concerned that the incident would call into question the rigor and validity of their food safety testing system. The biotechnology industry was concerned that the fact that the bacteria used were genetically engineered, which could be used as evidence that genetically engineered foods and drugs are unsafe. The food supplement industry was threatened because it was, after all, a food supplement that killed people.

❖ The most problematic ambiguity resulted from the fact that Showa Denko destroyed all samples of the genetically engineered organism as soon as the problem was recognized. ...Showa Denko had cut corners on the purification procedure used in producing tryptophan, and this occurred at about the same time that they began to use the genetically engineered bacteria.

❖ We conclude that it is likely the genetically engineering was the determining factor in generating this toxin."

VITAMIN A

Another common concern expressed by most beginning vitamin users is that "you can't take much vitamin A, because it can be toxic." Again, it solely depends upon your nutritional needs. In lands where there is severe malnutrition, it is not unusual for clinical doses of 100,000 IU's or more to be given on a daily basis for periods of several months. A very high fever in the course of some illnesses, such as scarlet fever, pneumonia or flues can rapidly deplete one's stores of A. Eskimos who subsist on whale blubber and oil in abundance, get very high amounts of this vitamin with no deleterious health effects. If one has a diseased liver, very large amounts in pill form should not be taken. Beta-carotene is converted to vitamin A in the liver. Diabetics and hypothyroid individuals are unable to convert beta-carotene to vitamin A. If one receives too much A (what would be considered toxic amounts) over a period of time, symptoms of a deficiency results. When the vitamin is stopped, the toxicity stops. It can be resumed at a later time in appropriate daily amounts. In general, it is suggested that pregnant women should avoid daily amounts over 25,000 IU and children taking A for more than one month should avoid amounts over 18,000 IU.   A nutritionally-oriented health professional can assist you in developing an appropriate supplement program.

B VITAMINS

Should you take an isolated B vitamin, it is a good idea to take it along with a B complex so as not to cause an imbalance in the body. Many drugs interfere with and decrease B vitamin levels in the body. When taking B3 (Niacin form), be aware that it may initially cause a "flush". A reddish, blotchy rash will appear on the skin at pulse points, on the back, face, extremities, etc., along with a feeling of hotness, mild itching and tingling. It will disappear within a short time and is a normal reaction.

Synergism, When To Take, How to Store

Vitamins and minerals are synergistic-- their combined effect exceeds the sum of their individual effects. When excessive amounts of certain vitamins or minerals are taken, this may cause an imbalance in other nutrients or interfere with the absorption of another nutrient. Common synergistic combinations are Vitamin C and bioflavonoids; Vitamin C and iron; Vitamin C and MSM (Methyl Sulfonyl Methane); Vitamin E and selenium; Vitamins A, D, and boron; Calcium, D, and boron.

In most cases, vitamins and minerals are taken with meals unless otherwise specified. Oil-soluble ones can be taken before meals and water soluble ones taken between or after meals. I think it is a good idea to store any oil-based supplements, such as essential fatty acids, in the refrigerator. Supplements should be stored tightly-closed in a cool, dark place, since sunlight and air decreases potency. Many of them have a expiration date stamped on the label, so be sure to check for it.

You have a wealth of many excellent books available describing the function and benefits of various nutrients. Remember, supplements are not drugs, do not mask symptoms, or work immediately. They should be just what the name "supplement" implies-- in addition to a good diet. They also can be used therapeutically to assist the body's healing capacity. When taking nutritional supplements and herbs, one should use common sense. It is not to your best advantage in health or pocketbook to "dabble" in taking supplements, but seek the good advice of your professional health care providers who know herbs and nutritional supplements intimately.

CHAPTER SEVEN

WASTE NOT! KEEP THE BODY CLEAN!

An old Indian saying goes,
If you want to see
what your thoughts were like yesterday,
look at your body today.
If you want to see
what your body will be like tomorrow,
look at your thoughts today.

From Deepak Chopra, "Journey Into Healing"

Waste Not, Want Not

Here's a new twist on that old proverbial saying. Keeping our bodies as waste-free as possible, that is free of toxic wastes of body processes, chemicals, pesticides, radiation, impure air and mental, emotional and spiritual wastes, we'll not be in "want" of good health. When our cells, tissues or organs begin to cry out for help by manifesting symptoms, we need to give them our undivided attention for healing to begin. It's time to clean up our internal and external environments.

Victims Unaware

We've hardly scratched the surface to identify the bombardment of environmental pollutants which occur on an unprecedented scale in our world today. We did, however, acknowledge the fact that we are often totally unaware of their presence. I cannot say that "totally unaware" statement without remembering one of the most pathetic offenses to the environment-- the world's worst nuclear disaster which occurred on April 25 and 26, 1986, in the Ukraine at Chernobyl. Untold hundreds of thousands of people had no idea there was a nuclear meltdown in progress until days afterwards. Thyroid cancer rates in Ukrainian children rose significantly in the years following this disaster. In the five years preceding the accident (1981 to 1985), the average thyroid cancer rate in children from birth to 15 years was 4 to 6 incidents per million. The years following, 1986 to 1997, the rate rose to 45 incidents per million. (10) Statistics never quite convey all the pain and sadness that accompany them.

Our communities are having to deal with toxic byproducts of routine industrial use that enter the atmosphere or are deviously and illegally being dumped. In cases like these, we may not be aware they exist until some investigation ensues and the media is brought in. Polychlorinated biphenyls are a good example. PCB's belong to a family of substances known as halogenated aromatic hydrocarbons. These are the some of the most poisonous chemicals known to man. They are released into the air by factories spewing dioxins and other carcinogenic substances from their chimneys. Dioxin is a byproduct of chlorine and shares gruesome company with DDT. These chemicals remain in the environment for many, many years, because they are extremely stable. PCB's are found in common products people use everyday such as pesticides, plastics, electrical equipment, paints, sealers, and adhesives. High-voltage transformers contain PCB's and also emit electromagnetic fields which, as previously discussed, have been linked to leukemia, tumors and other forms of cancer. Toxic chemicals may be dumped in the sewer system and find their way into the drinking water. There are accidental spills as well as purposeful dumping of toxic wastes into our oceans, lakes and streams.

Victimizing Ourselves

Other times we are responsible for our own pollution. Do we have any idea how toxic household and garden insect sprays are? Organophosphates, found in some pesticides, were used in the gas chambers during WWII, in the form of mustard gas, as well as the more recent Agent Orange herbicide used in Viet Nam. One of the problems

---

10) CANCER, Volume 86, Issue 1, 1 July 1999, pp. 149-156, American Cancer Society

lies in the fact that large chemical manufacturers are their own "policing agents", testing their products in-house and delivering the findings to the federal governmental agencies. It may take up to a decade of use before these products are found to be extremely hazardous and taken off the market. In the meantime, they inflict untold pain, suffering and possibly death to those exposed. These large corporations also finance tactically-arranged lobbying efforts to pass legislation restricting the rights of injured people. Thus manufacturers, insurance companies and other big business interests are successfully insulated from legal responsibility for injuries arising out of their carelessness and greed.

We need to be educated on what these can do to ourselves and our families. Pesticides can seriously damage our health-- kidneys, lungs, liver and many body systems and cause our death. Never forget, these are products are designer poisons-- *formulated to kill.*

Household cleaning products, aerosol sprays, napthalene-containing mothballs, toxic air fresheners, tobacco products, etc. are commonly used without any thought as to what they are doing to our health. When the fumes are detected, do we ignore them and assume they must be safe because these products are sold in stores? Is there some mental process that assumes we have galvanized stainless steel pipes for lungs and can breathe in anything unaffected? What about the products we use directly on our bodies-- makeup, skin care products, shampoos, conditioners, hair preparations? The packaging is skillfully contrived for impulse buying. Most of these products list their ingredients. How often do you read them to make an informed purchase? Perhaps you are thinking, "I don't really care. They make me attractive!" Actually, they're adding to the toxic stores that may be making you sick. All these toxins are cumulative. We are talking about substances that are known carcinogens or suspect of being toxic that are liberally used on our bodies each and every day. They all add up to burden our immune systems, can cause deep level tissue damage and deteriorate our senses. How often have you associated that headache, skin eruption, itchy patches, runny nose, frequent colds, nausea, etc., to the toxic overload in your everyday environment? Think about the composite amount of exposure from daily activities such as:

❖ pumping gasoline
❖ dry cleaning clothes
❖ sitting too close to the TV set,
❖ sleeping next to electrical outlets

 ❖ long periods in front of the computer monitor
 ❖ using electric blankets
 ❖ using hair dyes, nail polish, cosmetics with chemicals
 ❖ smoking, excessive drinking, drug use
 ❖ occupational and home exposure to heavy metals
 ❖ hobbies using toxic glues, solder, lead paints, etc.
 ❖ visiting nail salons and using acrylic nails (inhaling fumes
   and use of toxic chemicals) • unnecessary x-rays (They
   used to x-ray feet in new shoes years ago to see how they
   fit)
 ❖ over exposure to use of cell phones
 ❖ spraying pesticides
 ❖ use of anesthetics, drug residues
 ❖ using chemical products on our skin
 ❖ using toxic cleaning products
 ❖ using synthetic fragrances, preservatives, dyes, etc.

The World Health Organization blames environmental toxins for 60 to 80% of all cancers. Pesticides and other chemical pollutants which mimic human estrogen, are responsible for hormonal imbalances, dysfunctions, birth defects, still births, breast cancer and other cancers that are estrogen driven. As body tissues are saturated by toxins, minerals and antioxidants in vital body fluids are reduced or used up. Immune defenses become seriously impaired.

Free radicals from radiation as well as biochemical processes, cause us to age more rapidly and adversely affect the immune system. Heating fats changes the molecules to a carcinogens, and these we get through our diets. Free radicals can cause damage to DNA and the protective layer of fat in the cell membranes, cause retention of fluid in the cells and upset mineral levels. These free radicals are atoms or group of atoms that have at least one unpaired electron. Antioxidants such as SOD (superoxide dismutase), A, C, E, and trace minerals selenium and germanium can inhibit the formation of these free radicals by pairing up their free electrons. These antioxidants, help to detoxify the body by preventing free radical formation.

What can you do?

Implement changes in areas of living where you are in control Beyond that, become aware of the health hazards which exist in your community, county and state. Talk about these things to others you meet. Consider joining various non-profit groups actively educating the general public as well as legislators of the dangers to mankind and his planet. Search the worldwide web or your public library for "Non-profit Environmental Groups." Consider the important work they are doing on behalf of our rainforests, animals, sea life, birds, food safety, oceans, human race and other endeavors. Perhaps you may want to become a member to help support the work they are doing in preserving things precious to you and your family.

Our Bodies Self-Clean

One of the outstanding features of the amazing human body is a "self-cleaning mechanism." Our metabolic processes continually dispose of wastes and toxins. Keeping our organs of elimination healthy-- the skin, lungs, large intestine, kidneys, and liver-- should be a high priority. Ways that we can do this are by adopting the good health practices we have talked about in this book. Adequate exercise to keep our circulation sound and keeping stress under control are very important. Control our environment as much as we can individually and as families to lessen the use of toxic substances.

Colon Health

There's an old adage in natural health, "Death begins in the colon." It is crystal clear that poor bowel management is often the source of most people's health problems. Unfortunately, bowel management is not as hot a topic as time management. Especially in our culture, it is hardly ever talked about, even in the doctor's office. You may be told it's completely normal for you move your bowels once every four or five days.

Now, let me get real personal to make a point. I remember vividly years ago seeing a specialist for a chronic problem with constipation and hemorrhoids. After an extremely embarrassing colonoscopy (it happened to be a "teaching" day at the hospital, and my procedure was witnessed by a roomful of male interns; for those of you who are not familiar, you bend over a tilting table with derriere in the air as others stare. In retrospect, a collective mooning.) and minor surgery, I despondently asked him what I needed to do so that this situation would never happen again. Those questionable words of wisdom still ring in my ears: "Keep doing what you're doing. I can give you a prescription for stool softeners and hemorrhoidal cream. Once again, if what I had been doing was working, I wouldn't have had to go through that whole humiliating experience.

We've already discussed how each organ and tissue is dependent upon the well-being of every other organ and tissue in order to have total health. When there is faulty functioning in the bowel, the rest of the body is affected. How so? When a bowel is full of wastes and is sluggish, these wastes can be absorbed through the intestinal wall, into the bloodstream, and deposited in the tissues. This scenario impedes proper functioning in all body tissues where these toxins have settled. We're told to use laxatives or stool softeners when needed. These medications are not healthy as they draw water from the intestinal wall, pulling nutrients such as minerals in the process. Frequent use causes us to become dependent upon them, weakening our own peristaltic action. High-quality bulking agents such as flax seed, psyllium seed, triphala, and oat bran are a healthier alternative to harsh laxatives. They swell in the colon and act like a gelatinous plunger or broom to sweep it clean. It may take some time for this to occur, however, it makes a world of difference to your health. Be sure to drink lots of water and follow directions on the label or as instructed by your health care professional. There are a nice variety of high-quality products from which to choose at your local health food store.

In the past, people were far more knowledgeable on the importance of keeping the bowel clean and were taught how to care for it. Sufficient dietary fiber, fitting amounts of pure water, nutrients in the right amounts, healthy nerves, muscles and circulation are all important for bowel health. The typical American diet of refined carbohydrates, little or no fiber, insufficient water and improper food preparation leads to many bowel problems, especially constipation. Autopsies performed on some individuals have revealed an incredible accumulation of toxic waste, some occasionally weighing nearly 50 pounds! Though elimination may taken place on a daily basis or less frequently, this doesn't mean the colon is clean.

There are times when colonics or enemas may be appropriate. Colonics, also known as high enemas, should be performed by a certified colon therapist. There are two types of enemas. A cleansing enema will flush out the colon while a retention enema is held for approximately fifteen minutes to an hour or longer to replace intestinal flora or lost nutrients. Distilled water is preferable to tap water.

Host and Hostess With the Mostest

A dirty bowel can provide luxury lakefront living to very injurious bacteria and parasites. They attach themselves to the intestinal wall beneath layers of hardened feces to feed off of the nutrients that should be benefiting us and can live there a lifetime. They also can penetrate the intestines and travel via the circulatory system to anywhere they care to lodge and feed-- the eyes, brain, breast, liver, heart, lungs or elsewhere. As living things, they eat and excrete body wastes that are toxic to us. It is obvious they need to be addressed, for they are a constant drain on one's health and are often missed in regular health care. Routine laboratory tests are not 100% accurate in detecting parasites. In fact, the accuracy rate varies from lab to lab. Anemia, tiredness, clouded thinking, allergies, bloating, diarrhea, weight loss, gas or general weakness could be attributed to parasites. Healthy bacteria normally colonize the intestinal tract and are an important part of our natural defenses, keeping the bad bacteria in check. However, a one-time use of a potent antibiotic can wipe out most of the healthy bacteria. Antibiotics indiscriminately kill both the good and bad bacteria. After completing an antibiotic, it is important to replace these healthy bacteria. These are available in powder, liquid and capsule form. These friendly flora have such names as L. casei, L rhamnosis, B. bifidum, B. longum and L. acidophilus. There are also soil-based organisms (SBO's) which have shown to be an amazing breakthrough in healing and immune stimulation.

Worms are far more common in humans than most people realize. In America, they're a silent epidemic. Throughout the world, worms actually surpass cancer as man's deadliest enemy. Their sizes can range from single-celled, microscopic organisms up to 20-foot long tapeworms. Worms can impair or cause blockages in organs, often bunching together in a ball-like mass. Patients have undergone surgery for what was thought to be tumors, only to find these were actually "worm balls".   Even chemotherapy has been administered for tapeworm eggs in the liver which was erroneously thought to be cancer.

Fasting

Contrary to how it sounds, therapeutic fasting is not starving oneself. It is not wrapping oneself up in a loincloth and turban to become emaciated and jeered at in the town square. It is giving the body the rest it needs from eating, digesting and assimilating foods so energy can be channeled into detoxifying and repair. Rebuilding can begin as the body is cleansed and all the regulating powers are able to function without interference. If you fast from foods and only drink water for several days, your body will give you valuable feedback about your lifestyle. Some of the common cleansing reactions are headaches, fatigue, coated tongue, bad breath, body odor, achy joints, blemishes, diarrhea, mouth sores, and nausea, These are good to experience as they indicate that self-cleaning mechanism is engaged and working. A good detoxification program can be accomplished several times a year and should include cleansing. rebuilding and maintaining.

On a fast, the body decomposes and burns up only tissue and unwanted substances such as damaged, diseased cells, tumors, abscesses, fat deposits, and wastes. Eating nutrient-dense, raw whole foods, two days before and after a fast is important. We can ruin the desired effects by eating foods cooked, fried or smothered in fat. When it has been a proper fast for the right amount of time and broken correctly, all the body systems are improved to function at a higher level. Fasting should be accomplished along with a knowledgeable and experienced health practitioner who can monitor your progress. Avoid substances such as alcohol, caffeine, tobacco, white flour and sugars which are enervating; they lower or weaken nerve force and vitality. Continuing to eat nutrient-dense, living foods will help us stay at this higher level of performance. During the fast, get adequate rest, take peaceful walks outdoors, play beautiful music and read upbuilding material. As the body cleanses and the mind clears, a renewed desire to accomplish important things ensues. By modifying your lifestyle with healthy habits, the benefits of fasting will be longer lasting. Become empowered to know how you can keep your body clean through periodic detoxification and proper bowel management. Incorporating these natural hygiene methods will help you be much healthier.

More Waste of Another Nature

We are what we eat, digest, absorb and assimilate as well as what we think about, dwell upon, and sound down into our hearts. Toxicity can also come from the way we think and how we perceive both ourselves and our relationships in life. If our focus and our hearts are motivated by love, we experience the fruits of love, all contributors to good health. Conversely, a focus and heart motivated by hate begets sickness.

Every day we interact with people. We must function in relationships. Each individual grows on different levels at different rates, and for some growth is negligible. It's a fact of life that we find ourselves in the company of individuals who are toxic, not only physically, but mentally as well. They're miserable, unyielding, unthankful, disloyal, selfish, manipulative, angry, abusive and quarrelsome, obscene in behavior and speech. This "face" is not always obvious right away, as many times toxic people are cunning, clever and deceptive under the guise of spirituality. If your exposure to them happens to be in social circles, out in public or on the job, it is not too difficult to break the association. When it occurs in family relationships, we feel the ever-present smothering constraints and pain, affecting our health to a much greater degree. The weight is almost unbearable of ongoing negativism, irritability, belittling, unkindness, and unloving words and acts. There may be drug and alcohol addictions, sexual abuse, dishonesty, immoral behavior and a plethora of other offenses. These toxins impact us on all levels. We begin to experience the ravages of stress, headaches, sorrow, sadness, anxiety, anger, frustration, resentment and bitterness. The mind races day and night and the heart aches.

Do we succumb to a low self image, low self esteem, exactly what the toxic person puts out there for us to wear? Do we grumble and complain, and fight back adding more stress and pain to the situation? Do we feel that we somehow have contributed to the problem of this person "playing the victim" and feel personally responsible and guilty? Do we delude ourselves into thinking there is no problem because it's easier to pretend than deal with it? We need to supply some honest, soul-searching answers to these questions.

Allowing others to squeeze us into a mold of their perceptions, expectations and demands is not healthy. Love is sharing, nurturing, and allows for individual growth. An old Chinese proverb states: *God opens millions of breathtaking flowers each day without forcing the buds.* Others aware of the pain from our dilemma, offer counsel or advice. Becoming defensive when someone shows concern only perpetuates the self delusion that things are "fine". Sweeping things under the rug is not the answer. We are only as sick as the secrets we keep.

It is wise to seek professional help. We cannot be in the best of health while oppressive fears, doubts and emotions tear at our inner fiber. There are secular and spiritual counselors (professionals) who can give us practical guidance and wisdom. Yes, it takes courage to ask for help, and it takes great love to know that is what you must do. Fear paralyzes us and keep us from the healing we so desperately need only if we allow it. Relationships-- if they are truly worthwhile-- should enhance our health. They should, however, require us to grow so we know who and what we are. The rest of the healing and growth of the other person cannot be accomplished by you. You can offer help, but if not accepted, know what you must do to bolster your own strength, faith, immune system, inner convictions and inner peace. If the situation is abusive or putting you in harm's way, know that removing yourself from the relationship is the right thing to do. It is best not to "battle" to the very end in a fight that is not rightly our own. Sometimes that is the only thing that may wake up a toxic person. Lasting and enduring is not enough when the pain and suffering are devastating to your health.

A conscious effort to be waste free on the inside including body, mind and spirit will certainly bring our health to an exhilarating new high.   Never underestimate the powerfully detrimental effect that wastes and toxins have on the nervous system. Mental and physical depression, non-refreshing sleep, insomnia, excessive sleepiness, memory loss, excessive irritability, perverted moral feelings and insanity may be related to toxemia poisons. Remember, waste not-- want not.

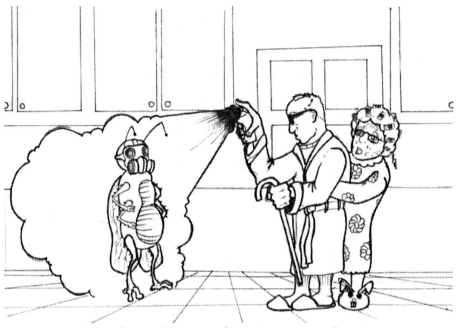

"I DON'T THINK IT'S WORKING, HAL."

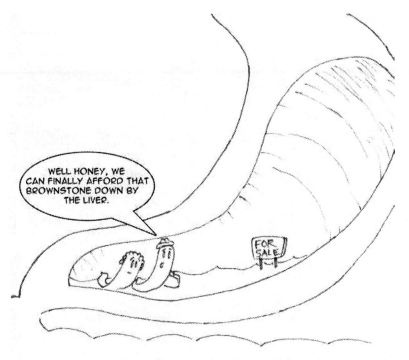

MOVIN' ON UP TO THE EAST SIDE

CHAPTER EIGHT

COOL, CLEAR WATER
AND PURE, FRESH AIR

*Drive across the Mojave Desert
in the heat of the day
without air conditioning.
I did. I appreciate water.*

Susanne

Cool, Clear Water

We drink it, bathe in it, play in it, swim and compete in it, travel on it, sing about it, enjoy looking at it, harvest food from it, and even give birth in it. Pure water is vital to life and is second only to oxygen in importance to health. Our bodies are largely made up of water-- close to 70%. Men's physical weight in body fluids is close to 60% while women who have more body fat are close to 50%. Infants have about 75% of their weight in body fluids. Our muscles are 75% water.

Water is biologically useful in allowing nutrients and chemicals of various kinds to be transported from place to place. Every cell requires water in order to perform its essential functions. It is necessary to maintain equilibrium, digestion and assimilation, and can be a shock absorber for joints, muscles and bone. It flushes out wastes and toxins, lubricates tissues, and hydrates the skin. Digestive juices are 98% organic water.

How Much To Drink?

Although we all seem to know how important water is to life, consuming adequate amounts of it on a daily basis is not the practice of most Americans. (Estimates are that 75% of Americans are chronically dehydrated.) Drinking between six to ten glasses daily under normal conditions is usually recommended. The body needs approximately three quarts of replacement water each day. If we engage in intense physical exercise, live in a more arid part of the country or in higher temperatures, we'll usually require more.

Most of us need a reminder to drink, waiting for our "thirst" signal to tell us. When you sense thirst, you've already waited too long as thirst is a signal of dehydration. You can tell rather easily if your water intake is insufficient by chronic constipation, hemorrhoids, varicose veins, dry mouth, skin, eyes, lips and nasal passages, fatigue, dark colored and/or strong smelling urine, frequent urinary tract infections, a history of kidney stones and regular use of diuretics. Diuretics, commonly called "water pills", pull water from tissues along with minerals, and increase the need for water. Many Americans prefer to drink beverages like soft drinks and sugary juices. Caffeine-containing soft drinks with high amounts of sugar or artificial sweeteners are counterproductive in replacing water loss because they also act as diuretics. On the flip side, there are some well-meaning individuals who will drink a dozen glasses or even gallons of water on a daily basis, feeling that this is healthy. It is the old "a little is good, so a lot must be better" mentality. This, however, is a bad idea since the body can become waterlogged and electrolytes are thrown out of balance.

When our family lived in the Southwest, my daughter came home from junior high one day and passed out in the kitchen. She had to run laps in gym class in the intense dry desert heat without being allowed to drink. Those in the fitness field especially should know you do not work out or do any strenuous exercise in the heat without replacing fluids. My husband, Jim, who has been in the fitness and nutrition fields for many years, met with her teacher the very next morning. That policy of no drinks during gym class was promptly changed. Sadly, some of our youth have died while participating in school sports due to a lack of proper hydration and electrolyte imbalance.

A Look at Quality

Considering the importance of water, we need to be concerned with its quality. We get our drinking water from two sources: surface water and ground water. Rain collecting in rivers, ponds, lakes, streams, etc. is surface water which municipalities use for our cities. Chemicals are added to it such as fluoride and chlorine to kill infectious organisms, and it is stored in reservoirs. Ground water is the source for rural areas coming from wells, springs and the natural underground aquifers. This is purified by passing through layers of rock and sand. Purified? Are these two sources pure?

Somewhere along the line, we inhabitants of earth considered the vast atmosphere surrounding the planet as well as our fresh water streams and deepest oceans as limitless dumping grounds. It's as though they have a never-ending capacity to accept all of the garbage, sewage, toxic industrial wastes, pesticides and other forms of chemical pollution. How far reaching is this problem? Our rivers and streams are becoming more and more carcinogenic, and underground aquifers are contaminated with toxic chemical pollutants and radioactive wastes. Most all the aquifers surrounding the nation's nuclear weapons facilities are heavily contaminated with radioactive waste. Worldwide, we hear of decomposing nuclear warheads and nuclear wastes dumped off the coasts of various continents as though they are "biodegradable". There are growing numbers of sewage landfills, toxic waste dumps and illegal industrial dumping yet regulations and enforcement of these are sorely inadequate. Many site operators, like ostriches with their heads buried in the sand, do not want to find out if substances are leaking because of the high cost to fix the problem. Shortsighted apathy?

The EPA lists some 48,000 chemicals yet only a small amount have been tested as to their effects on human health. Although over 2,000 chemicals have been identified in drinking water, most municipalities test for only 30 if they happen to have more sophisticated testing equipment. As a result, we find toxic chemicals, bacteria, viruses, radioactive particles, and heavy metals in the tap water we are supposed to drink. These pollutants can come from industrial complexes many miles away dumping toxic wastes that seep into our aquifers, lakes and streams.. From time to time we hear of deaths from cryptosporidium bacteria traceable to the drinking water. With such a sobering look at the condition of our water, it should move us to investigate better options.

Options

❖ Distilled water - natural spring or tap water is boiled and then recondensed (evaporation/condensation). Hydrogen and oxygen are left. Some water companies add minerals and ozone back into it.

❖ Artesian well water - water from a well in which water rises under pressure from permeable rock stratum overlaid by impermeable rock. It's source is deep, tapped by a drilled well. Depth, however, is no guarantee the water is pure. Pollution from twenty miles away or more may follow the aquifers and contaminate a well. My parents have a well close to 400 ft. deep. When tested from an independent laboratory, the water was unacceptably high in iron and had some contaminants such as E-coli.

❖ Sparkling water - from underground springs with natural carbonation (bottling companies generally infuse extra C02).

❖ Bottled mineral or natural spring water - The supermarket shelves have imported bottled water such as Perrier, Apollinaris, and Evian. Some commonly known domestic waters are Deer Park, Poland Spring, and Mountain Valley Spring Water. Water bottled in flexible plastic containers tastes like "plastic" and may not a viable, healthy option. The taste is indicative that plastic is leaching into the water, thus a pollutant. We have options to buy bottled water and have it delivered at home or office. Distilled water is preferable in glass and may be difficult to find. Most companies carry it in heavy plastic (Lexan) containers. Spring water is available in heavy plastic or glass. Ask your prospective suppliers for assays on quality.

There are also home filtration systems, distillers and purifiers. A reverse osmosis system with UV light to kill bacteria and parasites is effective. These systems remove bacteria, viruses, inorganic mineral salts such as fluoride, sodium and nitrates, heavy metals, organic chemicals, asbestos, dissolved minerals and particulates. They are not effective at removing toxic gases, phenols, some pesticides, and THM'S (tri-halo-methanes such as carbon-tetrachloride and chloroform).

Activated carbon filters are probably the least expensive and best method for removing foul odors, toxic gases, industrial wastes, pesticides, insecticides, chlorine, PCB's and THM's. These filters may also attract some of the heavy metals. Manufacturers sometimes forget to tell you that hot water may destroy the filter's ability to absorb and contaminants may be released from the filter. On the down side, they do not absorb inorganic mineral salts, have limited life and provide breeding grounds for bacteria. Chlorine, as we already touched upon, causes carcinogenic byproducts. The chlorine which was originally added to the water to kill organisms is filtered out, so bacteria, molds, yeasts and other microorganisms actually multiply unchecked inside the filter. If the cartridge isn't changed frequently enough, the backed-up bacteria will spill out into your glass in much higher amounts than you'd get directly from the tap. If there is a question about bacteria in the water, you can always boil it for about five to seven minutes.

Water distillers are the most effective at purifying water. The concept is similar to the evaporation/condensation method in nature--rain. They have distinct advantages in that the water is pure. It is colorless, odorless and tasteless. Some brands require that you periodically clean the stainless steel boiling chamber of mineral deposits that build up over time. There are some that are self-cleaning, and require maintenance once or twice a year. Be sure that the materials which come in contact with the distilled water are non-toxic, such as stainless steel or glass. The downside to distillers may be the price, rate at which the water is available, low yield compared to amount of water used, size of unit and use of electricity. The average time for an efficient distiller with a higher yield is about 2 and one-half to three hours per gallon. Since many brands do not eliminate toxic gases which may have the same boiling point as water, inquire about pre-boiling chambers and/or carbon filtration complements.

We should do what we individually can to conserve our precious water resource. Become proactive in stopping water pollution by buying non-toxic and natural biodegradable detergents and soaps. Stop putting chemicals down our drains and sewers. Use natural fertilizers and pest control in our gardens and use only what water we really need to bathe, shower, wash our vehicles and do our laundry. If not, the saying "water, water everywhere and not a drop to drink" may become a bleak reality.

> The forest leaves
> Convert to life the viewless air;
> The rocks disorganize to feed
> The hungry moss they bear.

Poem by J. J. McCreery

Pure, Fresh Air

McCreery's poem gives us a mental picture of beautiful trees of the forest filtering our "viewless" air. How painfully sad a large segment of the human race does not appreciate this unseen necessity to life-- fresh air-- or trees for that matter. The polluting of our air has been going on for centuries. Sure, in past civilizations, populations gathered around polluting wood fires in the wilderness. The problem is now that we have "progressed" to stripping the forests that filter our air to make way for more malls, factories and other profitable real estate projects. (Huge trees on the North American continent were being cut down for filler for toys, dolls and such by a large manufacturer in Japan.) Today we have progressed to aerosol cans, carbon monoxide from auto exhaust systems, pesticides, insecticides, smoke stacks of industry spewing out toxic wastes, and humans smoking like chimneys. Tobacco smoke contains over 4,000 identified poisons, any of which are lethal in high enough doses. That secondhand smoke contains lead, arsenic, carbon monoxide, cadmium and nicotine to name but a few. To show how dangerous nicotine is, it takes only one minute drop of pure nicotinic acid to kill an adult male. Nicotine is very addictive, but not beyond our ability to quit for our health's sake and that of others.

Years ago I recalled reading in a magazine how Russian children were being transported to clinics where they would be given "oxygen cocktails" because their city air was so polluted. Trendy restaurants and gathering places in America are now offering oxygen masks and oxygenating drinks.

Indoor Air

Even our buildings are sick-- the indoor air is far more polluted than outside air. The workplace can harbor deadly toxic molds and a build up of toxic chemicals due to poor ventilation. Windows are just for esthetic purposes rather than letting in fresh air. Air pollutants generally fall into two groups: gases of volatile chemicals such as paints, plastics, pesticides, and particulates such as molds, dust and pollen. What can we personally do to lessen air pollution in our homes and workplaces? Some practical things are:

- Use exhaust fans over gas stoves and ranges and make sure burners are properly adjusted.
- Stop smoking and discourage others from smoking in your home.
- Measure radon levels in your home and learn ways to reduce these levels.
- Make sure the crawl spaces and attics are well ventilated to prevent moisture and mold build up.
- Thoroughly clean and dry any water-damaged carpets and building materials to prevent the growth of molds and bacteria. These may need to be replaced.
- Use non-chemical methods of pest control.
- Choose paints which do not outgas harmful chemicals (such as Glidden Spred 2000 or AFM Safecoat).
- Replace pressed wood products and furniture when able with those that do not outgas formaldehyde.
- Clean carpeting with appliances that do not throw contaminants back into the air.
- Do not use chemical air fresheners or deodorizers and mask the air with petroleum-based fragrances.
- Change air filters in the air conditioning/heating system frequently and use a quality filter. (perhaps a few dollars more, but they are worth the extra money.)
- Stop using aerosol cans and switch to healthier, non-toxic products.
- Stop using office supplies with volatile ingredients.
- Read labels and become informed as to what pollutes and what is earth-friendly.
- Care about this planet by becoming a member of non-profit, pro-environment organizations.

If possible, consider air filtration systems and purifiers especially when their are known pollutants. Beautify your hom

ich are helpful in filtering the air such as aloe vera , spider
irysanthemums, fig trees, and English ivy. As much as
get outside during the day for breaths of fresher air. Take a
alk in the evening after dinner and talk. Take deep breaths and
appreciate the beauty of this planet. Get back in touch with the simple
things that are vital to life.

CHAPTER NINE

ENJOYING EXERCISE AND RESTFUL SLEEP

We find it is most ordinary
for people to be sedentary
working hard at desk and chair
and sitting home at night
to stare at television.
This isn't good for bones or heart
but exercise will do this part—
Play tennis, walk,
jump rope or run.
Exercising will be fun,
Just do it!

Susanne

Enjoying Exercise

"Exercise, me?" "You've got to be kidding." Is this what you're saying to yourself? If you think I don't understand and empathize with one depressed, chronically ill, overweight, out of shape, and feeling sick, believe me I do. I know firsthand what it feels like to walk a few steps, out of breath, and have limbs that feel like heavy rubber cylinders. Been there. Done that. I also made myself, pushed myself to get moving and get well. All the excuses in the world won't build health. Exercise is an integral part of the healthy living package.

A complete picture of health is obtained when we add all the pieces to the puzzle, so to speak. We may have a good diet and get adequate sleep and rest, but regular exercise is missing. Making changes to a healthy diet does bring very noticeable results rather quickly. Adding an appropriate exercise element, incorporating aerobic and strength training, you enhance appreciably anything done nutritionally. We'll become frustrated not seeing the results we want if we neglect any one area.

Benefits In Brief

There are numerous benefits I could list in regards to exercise and the body's biochemistry. Most of us know the obvious ones such as improved circulation, cardiovascular health, lowered blood pressure and heart rate, enhanced digestion and utilization of nutrients, a better outlook, increased bone density, weight loss, increased body tone, oxygenation to the cells and greater stamina.

Exercise keeps bones strong, muscles toned and flexible, blood vessels strong and healthy, and joints lubricated. If our muscles are weak, we are more likely to suffer back and joint problems and injuries such as strains and sprains. Stress is also a factor. Though exercise is a stress reducer and a good way to eliminate tension, anxiousness and depression, there is increased stress on the physical body. With this type of stress comes an increased need for high-quality nutrients, adequate rest and healthy eating habits. We're all unique biochemically requiring different nutritional programs, and each of us has special needs when it comes to exercise. Depending upon one's genetic make-up, health goals, fitness levels and limitations, it is wise to seek qualified help for an individualized exercise program. Most fitness clubs have certified personal trainers available to assist you and both in the club and at your home.

Exercise and Nutrition

Having worked with many exercise enthusiasts, athletes and members of health clubs, I have seen an amazing amount of people making unhealthy food choices with their exercise routines. Working out doesn't negate the need for optimal nutrition, but rather demands it. After all, the goal should not be to only "look good" but to enjoy vibrant health in order to accomplish one's goals and dreams.

Rewarding oneself with fast foods, beer, chemicalized, sugar-la
drinks, and sports drinks loaded with high sodium, chemicals
is not conducive to good health. Neither will gulping down
powders and bars in a base of sugar, chemicals, preservatives, etc. With
a level of mercury in every can of tuna, it wouldn't be reasonable to
ingest three to six cans daily as I have seen many do as part of their
daily protein intake.

One client, Ed, embraced the concept of healthy changes from the
start and would bring in all his snack wrappers from the previous week
to be sure he wasn't eating anything detrimental to his health. The
snacking soon gave way to wholesome, quality living foods. He could
not believe how much his stamina, performance and health had
improved.

An athlete or bodybuilder needs high energy, peak performance,
and endurance to compete. More calories are being used and replacing
them with empty ones serves no purpose. Rather, a regular, long-term
diet that's optimally nutritious is just common sense. Loading up on
carbohydrates before events or huge amounts of animal protein is
frequently done, but not to best advantage. Unrefined, clean-burning
complex carbohydrates from whole grains, whole grain pastas, beans,
rice, vegetables and fresh fruits are essential. Also, there are many
protein sources besides thick red steaks and tuna in cans. Fresh, wild
caught salmon and free-range or organic poultry are alternative choices.
High-quality proteins are also found in superfoods, beans, nuts, seeds,
whole grains, eggs, raw dairy products, and soy foods. Vegetarian
bodybuilders have proven that stamina, strength and good health are
not contingent on eating lots of red meat and other animals. Excess
proteins from red meats form toxic ammonia which burdens the
kidneys on excretion and can cause toxemia. Proteins from vegetable
sources are best for the absorption of minerals and bone density. So,
adjustments can be made to expand your choice of high-quality
proteins. Individuals with forms of arthritis have benefited greatly from
weight training exercise. Some have become bodybuilders and have
made incredible gains with professional help.

Getting Started

When embarking on any exercise regimen of your choice, it is best
to start slowly. Factor in time to stretch when getting out of bed each
morning. It is wise to start exercising two or three days a week to

gradually build up endurance. Make sure you warm up thoroughly by walking, jogging or bicycling. This will raise the body temperature and make muscles more flexible to prevent injuries such as tears, sprains and pulls. As the cardiovascular system becomes more conditioned, begin to incorporate strength training exercises such as free weights and/or weight resistance machines. By combining aerobic (cardio) and anaerobic (strength training) exercises, we see better results. When these two are not balanced in a program, we are more likely to over train and sustain injuries. Also, it's not "do more and faster" that will bring desired results. It's quality and form-- doing your routine correctly and enjoying the journey.

Oh, My Aching Body

A common complaint of people starting an exercise regimen is muscle soreness and/or stiffness. Much of that discomfort can be alleviated with proper warm up, cool-down and stretching. Waste products are produced while exercising-- uric acid, ammonia and lactic acid. These can form pockets of acid in the muscles and are very bothersome. A good massage along with some alkalizing foods will help reduce this natural result of exercise. Excellent alkalizers are raw fruits, vegetables and freshly-made juices. Homeopathic arnica is very helpful for strains, sprains or over exertion, along with ice/heat and rest. Arnica is also available in gel form to be used topically. An effective and safe natural anti-inflammatory for pain and swelling is bromelain taken on an empty stomach. Bromelain is a proteolytic enzyme which comes from the stem of unripe pineapples. It does not have the side effects of anti-inflammatory drugs. When taken with food, it serves as an enzyme to aid the digestion of protein. The body needs adequate rest in between workouts. (This doesn't mean years, months or weeks!) If any weight training is involved, don't exercise the same muscle groups two days in a row. Most people who are serious about exercise have made a practice of working out three to five times per week. They should alternate what they do at the gym each time, splitting up the muscle groups two days in a row. As already mentioned, it is very easy to overtrain, especially when you are getting started and your energy level comes up. I remember vividly those periodic fitness tests in high school. Everyone in class gathered around to count the number of sit-ups I was doing. Pushed to "greater heights" from the cheering crowd, I made it to 225. The next day, of course, I was unable to sit up or even move for that matter to get ready to school. Younger kids wishing to impress their friends may push a lot of weight around. Most often they are not exercising whole muscle groups by just picking out a couple of exercises they like. Muscle imbalance, injuries, dislocated bones, and muscle tears can be the result. These injuries may plague them the rest of their lives. There is also insufficient concentration on warming up and giving the body a chance to do heart rate recovery. It should be the goal of every trainer, teacher and athletic coach to be aware of the dangers in the gym and provide better instruction, supervision and involvement to those exercising, especially beginners.

Since muscles are mostly water, be sure to drink purified water often during your workouts. You'll need to replace the fluids you have lost, and don't wait until you are thirsty or cotton-mouthed. It is important to be re-hydrated through water, fruits and vegetables.

I'm too Busy

Perhaps the most common excuse not to exercise is "I don't have time." When your health is important to you, you'll make the time. Find something you like to do. Is it riding a bike, taking walks in the park, jogging, tennis, racquetball, swimming? If going to a gym or studio isn't your forte, there are exercise videos with quality training methods you can do at home such as Pilates, Callanetics, Taebo. You'll have to contend with more energy, flexibility, and a more youthful appearance. Can you handle that?

Life has its sleep,
its periods of inactivity,
when it loses its movements,
takes no new food,
living upon its past storage.
Then it grows helpless,
its muscles relaxed,
and it easily lends itself
to be jeered at for its stupor.

In the rhythm of life,
pauses there must be
for the renewal of life.
Life in its activity
is ever spending itself,
burning all its fuel.

This extravagance
cannot go on indefinitely,
but is always followed
by a passive stage,
when all expenditure
is stopped and all
adventures abandoned
in favour of rest
and slow recuperation.

Rabindranath Tagore

We're Best After Rest

Rest is necessary to de-stress, regroup and recharge from our pace of life. Work demands, family demands, financial demands, physical demands, all must be balanced with proper rest. When we take time out, meditate on upbuilding things, read a good book, listen to beautiful music, take a walk or sit in the morning sun, enjoy a therapeutic massage, hike through the woods to breathe the fresh air and commune with nature or sit at the beach and enjoy the ocean breeze. Whatever our preference, we should feel relaxed and refreshed after adequate rest. We need to schedule these times frequently for our health's sake.

Sweet Sleep

One-third of our lifetime is spent sleeping, a basic requirement for life. An average night of sleep for most people is 7-7 ½ hours. About

20% will sleep less than six hours and about 10% will average more than nine. It is important to get a sufficient amount of sleep to enable you to wake easily, maintain an alert mind, and enjoy life functioning optimally. Sleep is truly refreshing in a healthy lifestyle. It's that type of sleep where your head touches the pillow and you're out like a light. Many experiments and studies have been conducted over the years investigating and observing the sleep process. There are undoubtedly still undiscovered phenomenon relative to the process of sleep that will come to light in time.

Five Phases of Sleep

Researchers have identified five phases of sleep. During the first two and the last stage, the brain is awake. This is attested to by rapid eye movements, or REM. The eyeballs move about quickly in various directions beneath the eyelids as they would when you are awake. The brain is actually doing the "seeing" at this stage, while the eyes merely follow the images of our dreams. Blood flow to the brain is four times the normal rate during REM sleep.

Deep sleep lasts usually only 20 to 40 minutes, and in this stage the muscles are completely relaxed. The body becomes heavy and limp in one position, and the eyes hardly move. We partially awaken in and out of deep sleep allowing us to move about. This is important to prevent pressure sores from lying "paralyzed" as it were in one place. The heart rate and blood pressure fall and stabilize, while the brain's electrical activity shows a slowing down of regular activity. At this point we are as "dead" to our external environment. However, during the deep sleep phase, the restorative processes of the body repair and rebuild in adults and children experience growth as levels of the growth hormones rise.

When Sleeping Eludes Us

Nutritional imbalances, worry, stress, eating large meals before bed, parasites, family or work problems all are common reasons why we have difficulty sleeping. The purpose of going to sleep is to give the body and mind a much needed break for repair, refreshment and rejuvenation. Eating a heavy meal before bedtime causes the digestive process to work overtime. If we are harboring parasites, they usually get hungry or active about two to three a.m. They begin gnawing or can cause other intestinal unrest you may be feeling at this time. It's so common to hear, "No, I didn't sleep well last night. My mind was racing and I couldn't shut it off." Chances are you've been worrying throughout the day on the same issues, so give it a break and save the worry for another time. Better yet, realize that worry doesn't change a thing except contribute to your health decline. Do all you can to address the situation during the day, know your limitations in the matter and give it up to a Higher Source. Prayer works wonders to bring the peace that excels all thought.

Natural Enhancements to Sleep

Mineral deficits such as calcium and magnesium, may cause a drawing feeling in the calves and lower legs at night, sometimes called restless leg syndrome. Supplementing with these will help greatly.

Single herbs and herbal combinations are very effective sleep aids without the side effects of over the counter and prescription drugs. They are nutritive and will not bring that morning after grogginess or zombie-like feeling. Valerian, passionflower, California poppy, hops, lemon balm, kava kava and chamomile are some of the common herbs effective to help us sleep.

Pineal Gland and Melatonin

The pineal gland and melatonin levels are involved in the sleep process. The pineal gland is embedded deep within the brain and was named for its resemblance to a tiny pine cone. Like other parts of the human body, research has helped us to understand much about this gland, and much remains to yet be discovered. The pineal gland may play a role in stimulating the onset of puberty and is possibly the site of our biological clock-- the control center regulating daily rhythms such as sleeping, waking and keeping us in tune with changing seasons. Melatonin secretion continues until the interference from sunlight or full-spectrum lighting It makes sense to sleep in a darkened room and use a dim night light to see one's way clear to the bathroom so as not to disturb our sleep patterns.

Among other benefits, it is believed that melatonin slightly reverses shrinkage our master gland of immunity, the thymus, enabling greater production of infection-fighting T cells. It enhances antibody production and has antioxidant effects. Melatonin depresses the release of estrogen; risks for estrogen-driven cancers of the breast and prostate would likely be higher when melatonin levels are deficient. It has also been observed that when there is a sufficient amount of melatonin, the prostate decreases in size, just as a deficiency allows it to grow.

As we get older, like many other hormones, melatonin levels normally decrease. Rarely would it be needed in supplement form under the age of 40 except perhaps to counteract the effects of jet lag or an occasional sleeping disorder. If taken when not needed, sleep patterns may actually be disrupted. The supplement is a synthetic hormone which will have side effects like any other drug. These side effects can be in the form of decreased sex drive and shrinkage of the gonads. In fact, the reproductive system can temporarily shut down on high melatonin levels. Even the lowest dosage of the drug is considerably more than what we normally would produce. Hormones produced naturally in the body are extremely delicate, working in very minute doses yet powerfully impacting many body systems.

When taking synthetic hormone supplements like melatonin, DHEA, pregnenelone and others on a regular basis, the body tends to stop production of it own hormone. The literature accompanying these supplements suggest to have your doctor check your own levels first. Since long-term safety has not been determined with melatonin, it would be prudent to consider all the benefits and risks involved. If the decision is made to take it longer-term, a month or two break from it periodically may allow the natural production to resume.

A lifestyle combining regular, enjoyable exercise with restful, sweet sleep will certainly contribute greatly to being a more vibrant, energized and capable person.. If these two life-extenders have been escaping your practice, start today! It can begin with as simple as a brisk walk outdoors or if confined to bed, flex muscles, lift limbs, do whatever you can to challenge your body. When its time for sleep, relax, let the cares of the day go, and appreciate that you are pausing from all the physical activity, mental focus, and concerns to ref- let healing take place. Do not neglect these two importa- a healthy life.

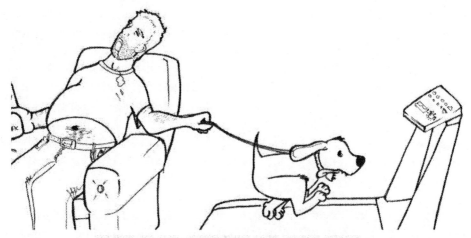

EVER SINCE GETTING THE TREADMILL,
STEVE'S BEEN GETTING LESS EXERCISE FOR SOME REASON

PART THREE: FEEDING THE SOUL

CHAPTER TEN:

HUMOR, LAUGHTER AND SONG

It's easy enough to be pleasant
when life flows by like a song,
but the man worth while
is the one who will smile,
when everything goes dead wrong.
For the test of the heart is trouble,
and it always comes with the years,
and the smile that is worth
the praises of earth
is the smile that shines through tears.

"Worth While" by Ella Wheeler Wilcox

Laughter, Good Medicine

Proverbs, a book of wisdom, in the 17th chapter, verse 22, says: "A cheerful heart is good medicine, but a crushed spirit dries up the bones." If you saw the movie "Patch Adams" starring Robin Williams, you clearly saw that health and healing call for positive thoughts and laughter. The cold, impersonal clinical approach of modern medicine has missed this fact all too often, and has received much criticism for it.

I did, however, manage an orthopaedic office some years ago in Allentown, Pennsylvania, and enjoyed a great number of humorous (as well as humerus) times. Even though it was serious business with four top notch surgeons, we easily could have been a TV sitcom behind the scenes. Good humor kept the stress levels down, and our patients actually enjoyed coming to see us.

We need to work toward wellness in a positive, determined way, and become empowered with accurate knowledge to accomplish it. Laughter is a blessing, especially when we can laugh at ourselves and laugh in the face of adversity..."for he who cannot laugh at himself, cannot laugh with others." We can feel its therapeutic benefits in the general sense of well-being. A hearty laugh relaxes muscles, and the diaphragm gets a good aerobic workout, increasing our ability to use oxygen.. Do you recall that "limp", euphoric feeling afterwards? Usually, you remember those situations that evoked the laugh for the rest of your life and tell those stories over and over again.

Serious Side of Laughter

Drs. Lee Berk and Dr. Stanley Tan of Loma Linda University, CA, have been conducting research on the effects of laughter. In students exposed to humor, they have evidenced lowered blood pressure and a reduction in stress hormones. Laughing triggers release of endorphins, our body's natural painkillers, and enhances immune function by increasing the numbers of antibodies. Interestingly, Drs. Berk and Tan found that subjects who watched a humorous video showed an elevation in immune activity which carried through to the next day.

Our family enjoys the tapes of Classic Carson Moments, excerpts from the Tonight Show. I'm especially fond of the animal segments. We also have tapes on the old Dean Martin Roasts. Every now and then we get them out and still laugh heartily. Good humor is timeless.... the Marx Brothers, Abbott & Costello, W. C. Fields, Lucille Ball, Steve Allen, Jonathan Winters, Charlie Callas, ---- and the list goes on. Feeling down? Put on a good comedy, and you'll be surprised how much better you feel. Ecclesiastes says "for everything there is an appointed time... a time to weep and a time to laugh." When was the last time you enjoyed a really good laugh? When we're take life too seriously day in and day out, it's not doing anyone any good.

Humor in My Roots

I am of Polish, Russian, Welsh and Cherokee descent, a Heinz 57 if you will. My Dad, Mom, sister and I lived in West Conshohocken, Pennsylvania until I was nine, and then moved to a little "farmette" of eight acres in Perkiomenville. Both my parents, Bert and Esther, have always had keen senses of humor that helped us get through everyday crises. Perhaps it had something to do with their growing up in large families. They taught me not to take myself too seriously, as I had a tendency to do that. In the midst of my fretting about something, Mom would just say: "It will all come out in the wash so don't worry about it." That would always bring a smile to my face. And, Dad is a study in persistence. When hitting a roadblock, he just finds another way to do it and whistles while he works. We called him "MacGuyver" because no matter what the need, he'd look the situation over then build or fabricate something with excellence to make it work. As a matter of fact, most of the relatives I grew up with were all very inventive and had great senses of humor.

Summertime meant huge picnics with family and friends that turned into marathons of sports, games, playing musical instruments and putting on elaborate amatuer shows. Wintertime brought the large ice skating parties, hot chicken soup and bonfires at our pond. Most of my uncles (Stosh, Pres, Alfie, Ed, and Joe) were self-taught musicians with tons of natural talent. I cherish all those times we played music together into the wee hours of the morning. Uncle Alfie was especially gifted-- inventing funny yet useful things, like a 3-foot long safety pin, wooden shoes with tops made from inner tubes (pre-dated flip-flops) and plaster of Paris heads from Halloween masks. He painted them to look like real people, and even gave me a haircut to put the finishing touch on one of his creations. (I can't believe I fell for that one.) His nickname "Morehead" was given him one day when his older brothers and a bunch of neighborhood pals were trying to figure out a solution to a problem. They labored over it for quite a while. When Alfie joined the group he asked what they were doing. When they told him the problem, he solved it immediately. They said he had "more head" than all of them put together. He was always the life of the party, always in good taste, and would have us all in stitches. As a matter of fact, he and my Dad did some carpentry work at Ed McMahon's home in Bryn Mawr, Pennsylvania. Ed asked him several times to come on the tonight show in N.Y. because my uncle was such a character. Uncle Alf never did take him up on the invitation. This upbringing helped me to see the "lighter" side of things in dealing with life's stressful situations.

A Hair-Raising Memory

One such stressful episode was the time I started a new job as Executive Secretary to a hospital administrator in Pennsylvania. I enjoyed walking to work rather than drive or take public transportation, about 14 city blocks total. This one morning the snow was coming down quite steadily and sticking, mixed with freezing rain, and the roads were getting slippery. My new boss called on the phone and told me he would swing by and pick me up due to the inclement weather. I thanked him for the offer, and decided to wear my brand new wig which I purchased for this type of yucky weather. As I climbed into his Mercedes, he complimented me on how nice my hair looked and commented that I should wear it that way more often. Again, I thanked him, patting my "hair" with my open hand as though to fix it better. We were on our way.

After parking the car behind our building, he suggested I walk ahead of him since the lot was becoming a skating rink. I carefully and daintily stepped onto the sidewalk with him following close behind. All of a sudden, my legs flew up in the air, I landed on my butt, my head jerked and my wig fell off! It wasn't enough that my own hair was "bobbi-pinned" tightly to my head, but my purse opened and it's contents rolled everywhere. I reached behind me without looking and frantically felt for the wig, forcing it onto my head. My boss let out a long, loud gasp, and after a quick "Are you all right?", hurried red-faced into the building. I gathered all my things with abject embarrassment and slowly headed to the front doors. How could I ever get through the rest of the day after this humiliating experience? As I caught my reflection in the glass, I saw such a funny sight I began to laugh hysterically. My shaggy wig was on backwards and stuck out like Woody Woodpecker in a windstorm. A mental picture of this episode invaded my thoughts throughout the day, and I could be heard cracking up with laughter in my office. My boss, on the otherhand, chose to play the recluse, too stunned to join in my bouts of laughter.

A Coat of Many Colors

Another time, I was going to Sunday service and noticed it was a bit chillier than expected. It was the perfect day to wear my new light blue, dress-length coat. I hung it in the foyer with all the other coats and proceeded into the main hall for some spiritual uplifting. When service was over, the sun was shining brightly and the temperature was considerably warmer. I grabbed my coat off the hanger, threw it over my arm and drove home. Monday morning, I was leaving for work and noticed once again, a light coat was necessary. In a rush, I locked the front door and hurriedly put on my coat heading to work. Part of my walk was on the main street of town where all the posh stores were. Everyone was all dressed up in their executive attire, and me in my new blue coat with my briefcase. Why were people staring at me? Not sure of what they were looking at, I caught my reflection in the large window of a department store.

"What is this?", I said out loud.

The hem of my coat was hanging down about four inches, all frayed on the bottom. As I turned to get a firsthand look at the back of my coat, I noticed a giant yellow mustard stain down the front of it with miscellaneous other stains of unknown origin. As a matter of fact, some buttons were missing, too. I had inadvertently taken someone else's coat that no one cared to claim for a long time. Same color, wrong coat. Again, I giggled and laughed all the rest of the way to work, with my coat of many colors over my arm.

A Humorous Look At Health

From READER'S DIGEST Condensed Version, comes "The History of Medicine":

"Doctor, I have an ear ache."
2000 B.C. "Here, eat this root".
1,000 B.C. "That root is heathen, say this prayer."
1850 A.D. "That prayer is superstition, drink this potion."
1940 A.D. "That potion is snake oil, swallow this pill."
1985 A.D. "That pill is ineffective, take this antibiotic."
2000 A.D. "That antibiotic is artificial. Here, eat this root!"

Norm Crosbys

The comedian, Norm Crosby, became famous for substituting the wrong word in his monologues. Over the years, people have said funny things (we call them Norm Crosbys) which we bring up every now and then and still get a laugh. I'll share a few with you on the subject of health:

❖ One elderly lady took me aside and in a quiet voice asked me if I could suggest some supplements for her husband who is impudent.

❖ Another who was trying to find B5 (pantothenic acid) and the mineral germanium, asked me for "pathetic acid" and "geraniums".

❖ A friend of the family said she called to get her medical records, but she had to wait because the doctor kept them downstairs in his "argyles".

❖ Aunt Ruthie was telling us her relative went in for tests since he had a pain right down here in his "Guadel Canal". (famous battle during WW II in the Solomon Islands, South Pacific).

❖ A neighbor was telling about someone she knew who had the "shaking palsy." My Mom offered, "Huntington's Chorea?" "No!" the neighbor said shaking her head. "She's from England."

❖ My all-time favorite was my parents' neighbor who had an extensive vocabulary, although she usually substituted the wrong words. Her brother had just passed away because he had " yellow janders." He was "so yellow he was green," and her son was a "ball-bearing" at the funeral.

We need to see the humor in things to lighten tension, stress and pain. It's part of keeping a healthy perspective and part of healing. I like the way it is beautifully put, in "Say It Now" by an unknown author:

> If you see the hot tears falling from a
> brothers weeping eyes,
> Share them. And by kindly sharing
> Own our kinship in the skies.
> Why should anyone be glad
> When a brother's heart is sad?
> If a silvery laugh goes rippling
> Through the sunshine on his face,

Share it. 'Tis the wise man's saying—
For both grief and joy a place.
There's health and goodness in the mirth
In which an honest laugh has birth.

The Joy of Singing

Unless you happen to be reading this while taking public transportation or sitting in a public library, I'd like you to try a little experiment. All right-- now think of one of your all-time favorite songs. Hopefully, you'll remember the words, but if not, humming will do. Sing it or hum it out loud, with feeling, as though you were auditioning for a Broadway show . Sing out like Barbara Streisand or Luciano Pavarotti. Go ahead, don't be shy.

Now, how do you feel? Relaxed? Upbeat? Calm and Peaceful? Energized? These are all good feelings or emotions. Remember the expression, "Music soothes the savage beast?" Perhaps most of the time you may not feel like singing, but try it. It helps. We all tend to get so overwhelmed with the day to day cares, that we forget to do the little things that inspire and uplift. A lilting tune or special song sung out loud has a wonderfully beneficial effect. My daughter and her good friend, Toni, have a ball with a karoke machine at least once a week. So, whatever music you enjoy, turn up the volume and sing your heart out.

I've quoted Eileen Caddy quite a bit throughout this book as she has written very concise and powerful inspirational thoughts. To end on a "happy note" from her book "God Spoke to Me":

"Let there be more joy and laughter in your living."

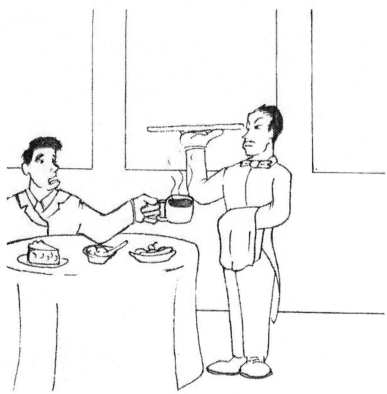

"DO YOU HAVE ANY SWEET-&-LOW?"

CHAPTER 11:

LOVE--THE MOST POWERFUL HEALER

*A bit of fragrance
Always Clings
To The Hand That Gives You Roses.*

Chinese Proverb

Mental, Emotional, Spiritual Health

A lifestyle to be healthy, must encompass not only the physical aspects, but the mental, emotional and spiritual aspects as well. Again, this is not considering mental health from a clinician standpoint, for that is a medical and chemical approach of which I have no expertise. But, I will talk to you from life experience. You don't have to be in "Who's Who" to know "What's what".

Each of us starts out in this human life without any prejudices, very trusting and full of love. We learn what we live, greatly impacted by the people around us in those early stages of development. Creeping into our learning processes are the contrasting philosophies and hardness of the world -- a contradiction of what we were as very young children. Growing pains bring introductions to strife and struggles, limitations, sickness, pain, addictions, obsessions, anger, guilt, oppression, corruption, greed, competition, prejudice, fear, anger, violence, selfishness and war. Values also begin to shift-- we may have been taught that having money and more material possessions than the next person is the objective, far more important than showing love. This perception of life is so empty and superficial since material things cannot love us back. Love cannot be displayed in a trophy case or parked in a driveway. It's feeling and healing energy given out to others. It flows out and returns to us. It is expressed in action through kindness, patience, humility, forgiveness, truthfulness, trust, hope, intimacy, and giving. As the wise proverb above reveals, the receiver is blessed by the gift as well as the giver as this is an act of love.

More Happiness in Giving

Each and every one of us has some special talent or ability, and sharing it with others doubles our joy. No price tag can be put upon it. Why is it we usually think in terms of running to the store to buy a gift that costs at least "so much" when its time to give something. Beautiful and meaningful gifts can often come in the form of intangibles. They can be sharing an experience that has taught us a great lesson, a clever and funny joke, a beautiful song, a funny story, words of encouragement at the right time, or deep emotional intimacy. A simple tray of wholesome, home-baked cookies with a little note saying how much you care can bring warm fuzzies. Share things like these with others.

Spending focused time with our children, listening to them, inspiring them, playing with and loving them is our precious gift. Phone calls to shut ins lifts their spirits and warms your own heart. Call friends to say "hello" and remind them how much you appreciate having them in your life. Even calling to say, I was just thinking about the time you did "this" for me. It brings back so many warm and tender feelings for both of you. Never underestimate the fun and excitement that comes with doing something in secret, when you see someone in need. Wrap up a box of something special with a big bow, put it on the doorstep, ring the bell and hide. It will give you a rush! Yes, the act of giving can cause your spirits to soar! I've always loved these two excerpts from "How to Be Happy" by an unknown author:

> Are you almost disgusted with life, little man?
> I'll tell you a wonderful trick
> That will bring you contentment if anything can,
> Do something for somebody quick!
> Are you awfully tired with play little girl?

Wearied, discouraged and sick?
I'll tell you the loveliest game in the world,
Do something for somebody quick!

Love is Patient

Sometimes we give our "gifts" and become disappointed when the reaction is far less than expected. Whether or not your gift is appreciated or accepted with grace, that very act of giving will gladden your heart. Realize, not every seed bears fruit, and sometimes the seed just takes a little longer to produce. I love how this is expressed in a poem penned by Edwin Markham, called "Outwitted":

> "He drew a circle that shut me out—
> Heretic, rebel, a thing to flout
> But Love and I had the wit to win
> We drew a circle that took him in!"

Thoughts and Emotions Affect Health

The physical aspects of health we have covered in other chapters. The mental, emotional and spiritual aspects are not in any way of lesser importance. Our attitude, outlook and spirit play an extremely pertinent role in health and happiness. Depression may be coming from a biochemical imbalance, a side effect from drug use, or other perhaps other causes. But, how we view our circumstances and life in general will help determine whether or not we progress towards healing. We need to conquer bad habits and deal with life's stresses in a healthy way. By turning away from love we experience frustration, hardships and pain. Remember, grief is halved, and joy is doubled.

Yes, by worldly standards, "we've arrived" when we reach an apex in ego with a matching monetary bracket. It seems to spawn a mindset to look out for number one, and too bad if someone gets in the way. Using others for selfish gain, is hardly "arriving". We really arrive when we tap into the bigger picture of life, surrender to a God of love, and let Him direct our lives. That Love redirects us away from all the disagreeable and ugly things the world has taught us. We may not perfect it now, but we can move ever closer to it. There is more than enough bleakness on the evening news and in the daily papers. Sometimes, these great hardships and tragedies touch us personally. It is very difficult for anyone to keep giving out without replenishing one's own stores. We need to be disciplined to spend time in good company, good books, and with those who can inspire us to use our gifts and talents in the service of others. Plan some volunteer time even in a very busy schedule. You'll reap wonderful benefits.

Expressions of Love

When it comes to health, I often think of many individuals I knew personally who were suffering with what were considered terminal conditions or challenging physical handicaps. What lights they were. After being in their company, I would be so uplifted.

Charlie especially stands out in my mind. He was a quadriplegic who lived in Good Shepherd Home in Allentown, Pennsylvania. His name was given to me by a friend who wanted me to visit and encourage him. I prepared for several days wanting to be sure I'd have a head, heart, and basket full of good things to share. I happily made a trip to the Home, and hoped Charlie would be available for a visit. An employee led me down a long corridor, not to a room as I recall, but to an area that jutted off the main hallway. I was quickly introduced to a man who was confined to his wheel chair. In order for him to look up and speak, it took a great deal of effort to lift his head and try to control his neck muscles. When he spoke, it took extra concentration on my part as he thrust out his tongue to utter the words. I noticed he was sitting in his chair at a little table with a typewriter. Guess what he was doing. He had a band on his head with a little hammer that would pound an individual key on the typewriter. He was busily writing letters to encourage families mentioned in the newspaper who had just lost loved ones-- one stroke every minute by using his head. That brings tears to my eyes as I'm writing this. I was the one so privileged that day, the one who came away encouraged by the love in that beautiful man. I left very thankful for all that God has given me. When we give to others, we give to ourselves and what we withhold from others, we withhold from ourselves.

We need to take responsibility for our thoughts and actions. We can go around blaming everyone one else for why we are the way we are, but the truth of the matter is that we have a "choice". One of my all-time favorite poems is called "MYSELF" by Edgar A. Guest:

I have to live with myself, and so
I want to be fit for myself to know,
I want to be able as days go by,
Always to look myself straight in the eye;
I don't want to stand, with the setting sun,
And hate myself for things I have done.
I don't want to keep on a closet shelf
A lot of secrets about myself
And fool myself, as I come and go,
Into thinking that nobody else will know
The kind of man I really am;
I don't want to dress up myself in a sham.

I want to go out with my head erect,
I want to deserve all men's respect;
But here in the struggle for fame and pelf
I want to be able to like myself.
I don't want to look at myself and know
That I'm bluster and bluff and an empty show.

I can never hide myself from me;
I see what others may never see;
I can never fool myself, and so,
I want to be fit for myself to know,
Whatever happens, I want to be
Self-respecting and conscience free.

CHAPTER TWELVE:

SHARE THE HEALTH

My wife was very sick so we called Dr. Griffin.
He gave her some medicine and she got worse.
I then called Dr. Kurth and he gave her some
more medicine and she still got worse.
I thought she was going to die, so I called Dr. Cross
and he was too busy, and finally my wife got well.

From Bob Phillips' "Good Clean Jokes"

Our Right to Choose

Health care providers should be highly-qualified in their respective fields. They should teach us how the human body functions and offer opinions, options, answers, courses of treatment, remedies and intelligent, appropriate therapies. The decision to follow this advice is yours. We should never be intimidated by disease or the caregivers for it. With something so precious are our lives, how can it be beneficial to be rushed ahead by fear and intimidation. An appreciation for the whole person including the mind, emotions and spirit is left out. When that is the case, hindsight usually brings wishes that we had taken another route. The process of getting well should be a "sharing" process. It has to sound and feel right before we proceed. We should feel that everything presented to us is the complete picture as far as possible, and then we can move ahead confidently and positively to our goal. After all, who has the highest stake in the outcome? We owe it to ourselves to find out all we can about what condition we are addressing. There may be times when our health concerns warrant a second, third or fourth opinion from qualified health professionals. No competent practitioner in any field should be offended if you seek another opinion. To illustrate, if you take your favorite garment which has a visible stain to someone who only has a pair of scissors, in all likelihood the stain will be cut out. Upon seeking another opinion, you are told how to get rid of the stain while leaving the garment intact. A more appropriate tool or method accomplishes the task with much more favorable results. You realize no one can build health but you by supporting that incredible healing ability within.

Holistic Nutrition

The principles of natural health can be learned readily by any student desiring a lifestyle that empowers us to greater energy, vitality and peak performance. They are common sense, practical approaches to everyday living. Holistic nutrition, on the other hand, actually is a specialty all its own. Don't blame your medical doctor for not applying a vitamin, mineral, diet, exercise approach to his/her practice. Even if they wanted to, most busy physicians simply don't have time to learn what is in effect a whole new orientation and specialty. They are highly trained in diagnosing illness, prescribing drugs and performing surgery. Their training demands the study of drugs-- their applications, contraindications and interactions. Nutritional information in medical schools has routinely consisted of about 3 classroom hours, which hardly scratches the surface of learning what nutrients we individually need biochemically to get back into balance.

Keep Your Senses

You'll sometimes hear from doctors a cautionary warning that nutritional therapy is dangerous because precious time is wasted. The condition will be too far gone before regular treatment is given. How can changes that build health be detrimental to it? Any health care provider who sincerely has the patients' best interests at heart should do everything possible to insure this does not happen. The whole purpose of health care after all is to keep people healthy and help the ill return to health as timely and safely as possible. Thomas Edison's insightful quote is worth repeating:

"The doctor of the future will give no medicine, but will interest his patients in the care of the human body, in diet, and in the cause and prevention of disease.

Whoever you choose to work with you as your health practitioners should firmly believe in the concept that you are personally responsible for your own health. They are there to provide you with the education and tools necessary to build and maintain health. You are the one who does the work, makes the changes and sees the results. I mentioned early on, it is the desire, education, commitment and personal application that brings results.

Don't forget to check your local area for suppliers of high-quality supplements and fresh produce, preferably organic. If you choose to eat meat, make sure it is hormone-antibiotic-chemical free, either free-range or certified organic. For further assistance, please visit my website at www.naturalhealthchat.com. This features an interactive site for one-on-one consultations and other options such as upcoming lectures, a mailing list and innovations in natural health. I look forward to your comments or questions. Also, please let me know if you found this book to be helpful to you.

PSYCHIATRIST

Patient: Every night when I get into bed I think that someone is under my bed. I then get up and look. There is never anyone there. When I crawl under the bed and lie down, I get the idea that there is someone on top of the bed. I then get up and look and I never find anyone on top of the bed. This goes on all night, up and down; it's driving me out of my mind. Do you think you can help?

Phychiatrist: I think I can. All you have to do is visit me twice a week for the next two years and I think I can cure you. The visits will cost seventy-five dollars an hour.

Patient: That is an awful lot of money for a working man like me. I'll have to talk it over with my wife and let you know.

The next week the patient phoned the psychiatrist.

Patient: I won't be back doc. My wife solved the problem. She cut the legs off the bed.

(From *The World's All-time Best Collection of Good Clean Jokes*
by Bob Phillips)

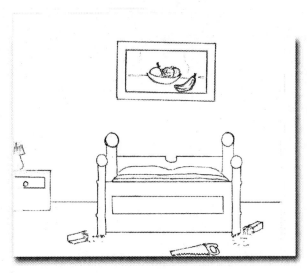

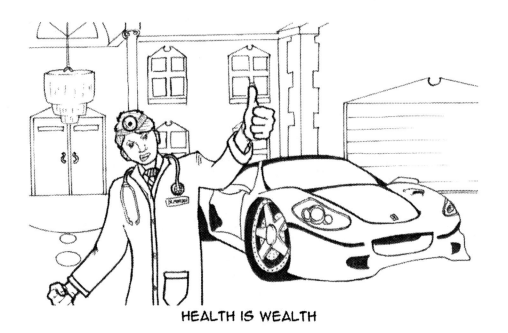

HEALTH IS WEALTH

Closing Remarks

It doesn't interest me to know where you live
or how much money you have.
I want to know if you can get up,
after the night of grief and despair,
weary and bruised to the bone,
and do what needs to be done
to feed the children.

Oriah Mountain Dreamer in "The Invitation"

What power in these beautifully written words of Oriah Mountain Dreamer. She creates a mental picture of struggles, hardships and sheer will that touch my heart in a special way. We as grown-ups, whether parents or role models, have a duty to show our children by example the "stuff" we are made of-- determination, fortitude, integrity--by doing what needs to be done in spite of heavy burdens. Children learn what they live, depending on us for so much. They view us as the measuring rod for how to live.

Today it is not only the adults who are facing unique challenges. Our children are gripped by fear, uncertainty and decaying moral values penetrating their worlds. To rise above whatever trouble each new day brings, we must take care of ourselves and we must also "feed the children." We must feed them physically not with junk but with life-sustaining, beneficial nutrients and feed them spiritually with principles to last a lifetime. Is there one common denominator that holds the key?

I guess it all boils down to appreciation. When the tough-going gets tougher, we have to know where our treasure lies. I know with every breath I take and every ounce of life in me, that we can choose a path to follow that is life-saving. We can choose health by how we think and live. The bottom line is being honest with ourselves, humbling ourselves and asking how we fit into the greater scheme of things. We must never stop questioning, recognize practical wisdom and safeguard our thinking ability. We cannot peer into the depths of outer space, examine a delicate flower petal under magnification, or gaze at the splendor of a magnificent sunset without evidence of Divine order. Look around you and see the stroke of the masterful hand of an incredibly Awesome Creator. He genuinely cares about what happens to each of us. He's made provisions for everything we need to live in health now, and forever. I encourage you to seek Him out in prayer, and search His written Word for answers. Be blessed!

Susanne/ 2003

Printed in the United States
26676LVS00008B/103-120

9 781932 560831